Anxiety | Depression | Trauma

BREAKING
THE
SILENCE

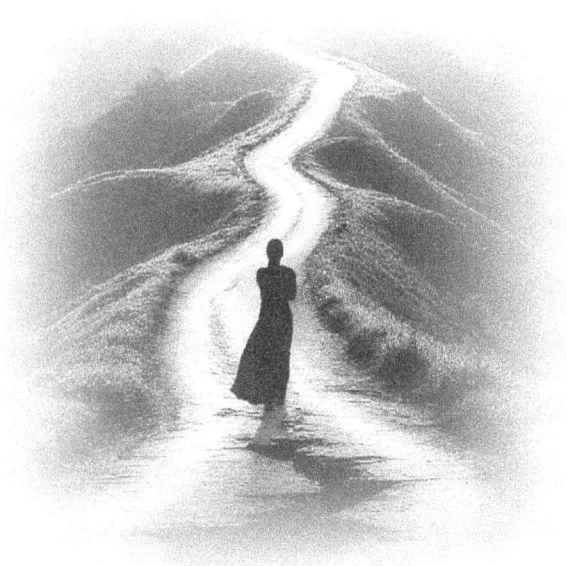

BOKALI CHISHI MUGHAVI

Dedication

This book is dedicated to
Iza Kheholi Chishi, Ingu Piwoto Chishi & Ingu Shikato Chishi

Endorsements

Breaking the Silence does exactly what the title promises it will do. Suffering is often destructively silencing. It closes us down and separates us from our ability to even articulate the pain. Bokali Chishi Mughavi courageously and powerfully shares her journey through these tangles and excruciating experiences and, in so doing, breaks the silence and points toward hope and redemption. This is a life-changing read.

David M. Goodman
Ph.D., Dean of the Woods College of Advancing Studies at Boston College, USA.

In *Breaking the Silence*, a deeply inspiring memoir, in which Bokali shares her journey through the depths of mental illness, revealing how unwavering faith in God became her lifeline. Through the darkest moments of anxiety and despair, she discovered the liberating power of trust in Christ. Blending raw vulnerability with spiritual wisdom, this book offers hope to those facing similar struggles, showing how faith combined with medical help can lead to healing, peace, and a renewed sense of purpose.

Dr. John Varughese
Dean of Doctoral Studies and Dean of Students.
South Asia Institute of Advanced Christian Studies (SAIACS), Bangalore.

Talking about mental health is imperative to reduce the existing misconceptions and stigma and also encourage those suffering to seek help and find support. In this book, Chishi bares her soul to shed light on the nuances of mental illness, the symptoms and patterns in the family system and the changing environments. With wisdom and profound personal experience, Chishi guides us to identify, face and process pivotal moments of life that makes up the long painful journey of understanding mental illness.

Every chapter is imbued with compassion for brokenness as well as appreciation for each new opportunity life brings. Chishi offers thoughtful and honest explanations of the depth of human brokenness as well as a big picture of such manifestations and ways to embrace new knowledge and persevere, thus breaking the patterns of the illness. Reading this book will help one understand the various aspects of mental health, and give care to those suffering from illnesses as well as to the caregivers.

I highly recommend it.

Rev. Dr. Ellen Konyak Jamir
Dean of Students and Associate Professor of Pastoral Counselling and Psychotherapy at Oriental. Theological Seminary, Bade, Dimapur, Nagaland.

I have known Mrs. Bokali Chishi Mughavi since 2004, and together, we have served diaspora communities since then. Her dedication to helping people in South Korea and Nagaland stands as a powerful example of how God can work through small yet growing mission efforts. In *Breaking the Silence*, she shares her inspiring journey, showing how God can use humble and faithful servants, regardless of their resources, to achieve great results for His glory. He reveals his redemptive plan and reconciling work in the world regardless of time and events.

Rev. C.S. Barnabas Moon
Lead Pastor, Living Hope Church
Director, WiThee Mission International
Executive Director, Korea Evangelical Fellowship Mission Commission
Professor of Intercultural Studies, Jeonju Vision University, South Korea.

Published by

Maurice Wylie Media

Your Inspirational & Christian Book Publisher

Based in Northern Ireland and distributing around the world.

For more information visit

www.MauriceWylieMedia.com

Publisher's statement: Throughout this book, the love for our God is such that whenever we refer to Him, we honour Him with capitals. On the other hand, when referring to the devil, we refuse to acknowledge him with any honour, to the point of violating grammatical rules and withholding capitalisation.

Contents

SECTION 3: EMBRACING THE FUTURE
Wrong Thinking Equals Wrong Results

Foreword

When you've taught someone for several years, you might assume you know them well. But I was wrong. You've probably heard the saying, "You can't judge a book by its cover"—how true that is! Boka, as she is affectionately known, was my student for three years during her Master of Divinity programme at Oriental Theological Seminary. I thought I understood her well, and to some extent, I did, but it was mostly based on our student-teacher relationship.

Boka was exceptional in her studies and consistently outperformed her peers. I believe she could have achieved even more if not for her health challenges. She often needed to leave class for medical check-ups, and I was aware of her struggle with frequent nosebleeds, but she always composed herself admirably. Despite her difficulties, she persevered and succeeded. She is indeed a strong lady.

Our cordial relationship developed further beyond her student days and has continued into her married and family life. I've come to know not only her children but also her husband, Major Dr. Mughavi Y. Sema, a man who loves the Lord and his family deeply. Boka once reflected, "It's amazing to see how far I have come and where I am now. I am truly thankful to God."

Reflecting on Boka's journey, I am struck by the inner strength and determination that have brought her to where she is today. Imagine yourself in her shoes. I don't think most of us would have made it through. Very few people truly grasp the complexity of mental illness, and even fewer dare to talk about it. The stigma which society attaches to this illness is overwhelming. It's one thing to struggle privately; coming out publicly is something entirely different.

In Nagaland, mental health struggles are still often kept as family secrets. Only the strong speak out, and only the brave share their stories. It takes immense courage to open up about something so deeply personal. Those who do often face judgement, suspicion, and misunderstanding from others. Most people choose to remain silent to avoid further criticism. But when someone like Boka decides it's time to share, it can create a ripple effect, often a positive one at that.

The life story and journey shared in this book are eye-opening. At every turn, you will find yourself asking, "How did she make it through?" Boka's ability to endure so much reveal a strength that only comes from allowing God to take the lead.

Boka trusted God through the darkest seasons of her life, transforming them into a vibrant testimony of victory. This is not a mere religious attribution; it is the testimony of genuine faith that saw her through her dark seasons. God was her source, and the Holy Spirit persistently worked in her life through the prayers of her mother. God did not give up on her because neither she nor her mother gave up on Him.

This part of her story may not resonate with everyone, especially when reading about the little four-year-old girl who endured so much until adulthood. One can only imagine the labels and silent stares she endured from those who judged her from the sidelines. But what she clung to, her belief in God, sums up everything she now calls *Breaking the Silence*.

There is one message that stands out: there is hope. Hope for those who believe and persist. The author's reliance on God and her deep spiritual conviction has been her true anchor in overcoming these dark moments. The trauma people endure with mental illness is something we have ignored for far too long.

It's not just the individual who suffers, it's the whole family. This is why the need to address mental health is critical. We must educate our people, from children to elders. We must join Boka in speaking out and addressing the issue from all angles, including the spiritual realm. Family, Church, and community all have roles to play, and this book must lead the way so that we can confront the issue head-on.

I thank the writer for taking this bold step. She has done a great service to the Church and humanity by sharing her story. The author's success is also the success of her husband and children, who walked through the ups and downs with unwavering support, offering help and guidance to where she stands today. *Breaking the Silence* is a must-read for those facing dark moments in their lives and for anyone seeking to understand how mental illness affects people and how we can reach out to them.

As you read the pages of this book, may you find inspiration and strength, just as the author has shown us how to face life positively. May we, too, break our silence, speak out, and stand up for those journeying through fear and pain.

Thank you, Boka, for sharing your story. I am blessed and determined to speak for those whose voices are not heard.

Rev. Dr. Zelhou Keyho
General Secretary of the Nagaland Baptist Church Council (NBCC).

Introduction

I was shocked when I read the World Health Organization[1] (WHO) World Mental Health Report (2023), that a staggering one billion people (more than one in eight adults and adolescents) worldwide have a mental disorder. Depression (280 million people) and anxiety (301 million) are the largest groups, but also developmental disorders, attention-deficit hyperactivity disorder, schizophrenia, bipolar, and conduct disorders affect millions of people across the globe with mental health conditions. I then learned that the Indian state of Nagaland, where I am from, might have an even higher ratio. This finding was a wake-up call to me and of personal concern. It's not just about numbers—this is about our lives, our futures, and our hope.

Delving into it more, I discovered that the most common mental illnesses in our state are schizophrenia, mood disorders, depression, anxiety, and substance-related disorders. The rising use of cannabis among young Nagas is exacerbating the problem, taking our young lives, and stripping our precious state of its future generation.

The question is, what are we going to do about it? Will we sit idle and watch our children fall into addiction, leading lives devoid of peace, joy, and our Naga values? Surely not. We are better than that.

With this in mind, I have decided to share my experience, revealing the dark journey I have endured, the fight to be whole, and the light I now embrace. If God can do it for me, then He can do it for anyone, including you and your family.

I was only four years old when I was first exposed to mental illness. Fear took hold of me that day, with stress, torment, and sickness following. I had now stepped into my uncle's footsteps. Mental illness wasn't just another word in our family; it was something very real,

---

[1] https://www.cambridge.org/core/journals/the-british-journal-of-psychiatry/article/who-world-mental-health-report-a-call-for-action/D0DC7D90FD2CF0D6199D6D90C0F662E1

lurking in the corners of our minds and souls until God showed us the keys to freedom.

I was raised in the state of Nagaland, located in the north-eastern region of India, a small, hilly state that visitors often call the 'Switzerland of the East' because of its beautiful mountains and green hills. In a Christian state, most of our churches are filled with people each Sunday and our largest church has a weekly attendance of 8,500[2] people.

Then one might wonder, why do we suffer from so many mental health issues? Is it possible that there is a disconnect between the teachings of the Bible and our daily lives as Christians? One of the many lessons I have learned on my journey to wholeness is that we must surrender daily to Christ, and in doing so, He will fill us with understanding. God wants to lead us to a promised land of peace and a sound mind. But how can we achieve this when negative seeds are constantly being sown?

We must understand and deliberate carefully: we become what is sown in us.

When I was young, I visited my maternal uncle who lived with my grandparents. The shock of seeing him for the first time, and the subsequent visits, planted a deep seed of fear in me. It wasn't just fear of him but fear that I might become like him.

Children are like sponges; they absorb everything, whether good or bad, for they do not know the difference. That is why we, as parents, must monitor what they see, hear, taste, and do. My parents took good care of me, but they didn't realise that such exposure could harm, or rather, damage me.

My uncle was suffering from severe mental illness, and to prevent him from hurting himself or others, he was kept chained at my grandparents' house. They used terms like 'mental problem' and

---

[2] https://en.wikipedia.org/wiki/Z%C3%BCnheboto_S%C3%BCmi_Baptist_Church

'demon-possessed' when referring to him. He was very violent and hostile, and although it was heart-breaking for my mother's family, keeping him chained was the only way to ensure everyone's safety.

At that time in Nagaland, there were no proper psychiatric wards in private or government-run hospitals, except for one mental hospital run by the state government, which lacked high standards. In 2010, the Christian Institute of Health Sciences and Research (CIHSR) in Dimapur added a mental health wing to its facilities and initiated awareness programmes, quite a significant step towards supporting people. Individual counsellors and therapists are also contributing by creating awareness on social media and other platforms. Some mental health professionals and NGOs have started counselling centres and are working to raise awareness about mental and emotional wellness.

When my parents and I visited my uncle who had been admitted to a mental hospital in Assam, the neighbouring state of Nagaland, for proper medical treatment. I remember seeing my mum and her sister cry every time my uncle was taken in for his treatments. Though my memories are hazy, I distinctly recall their conversations and sobs about the "electric shocks" [3] as they waited outside. Growing up, I often wondered what the treatment was all about. However, I never dared to ask my mum about it.

It was only when I became an adult and visited the doctor that I began to understand the questions many of us are asked. The doctor would inquire, "Does anyone in your family have this condition?" or "Did your parents or grandparents have it?" They were searching for the thread, the connection, or what the Bible explains as 'iniquity', something that has been passed down to the next generation.

I was starting to feel fear gripping me, and at times, it would overcome me. But where was its source or strength coming from? I was about to find out.

---

[3] Known as Electroconvulsive Therapy (ECT). According to the Mayo Clinic's website, "ECT is a procedure done under general anesthesia in which small electric currents are passed through the brain, intentionally triggering a brief seizure. ECT seems to cause changes in the brain's chemistry, which can quickly reverse symptoms of certain mental health conditions."

My mother had suffered a series of traumatic events. She lost three of her nine siblings to mental illness, one after the other, over a decade and a half (from the early 1980s to the mid-1990s). While all nine of them are still alive, three of them have never fully recovered. I witnessed my mum, the oldest of all the siblings, go through untold pain and grief. But I was not aware that I, too, would face this unbearable condition, which we now know as Post-Traumatic Stress Disorder (PTSD).

At that time, I lacked the awareness and tools to cope with the pain that my body and mind were experiencing. I suffered immensely, never imagining I would find any form of help, healing, or restoration. With everything taking place, how could I deny them?

I did not know then that my immune system was weak, which made it difficult for my stomach to retain solid food. This led to various allergies and infections. Despite my physical health issues, I grew up like any other normal teenager until I was 19 years old. At that age, all the bottled-up, unprocessed pain, anger, fear, and other unexplainable emotions began to surface in my head, heart, and body. I felt like I was about to explode, without understanding why.

The underlying cause of many of my health problems was my lack of spiritual understanding. The Bible says, "*The truth shall make you free,*"[4] yet I was in complete bondage. It also says, *"And I will give you the keys of the kingdom of heaven, and whatever you bind on earth will be bound in heaven, and whatever you loose on earth will be loosed in heaven,"*[5] yet I felt powerless. This led to an anger problem with God. I struggled with expressing my anger at Him for the helplessness I witnessed around me, which brought many questions in my mind. I saw my mum and her siblings lose two brothers and a sister to mental illness. I felt ashamed when our family friends asked about my uncles and aunt, questioning why they lost their minds. These questions remained in the back of my mind, strengthening the seeds

---

[4] John 8:31-32.

[5] Matthew 16:19.

of helplessness growing in my soul.

In September 1997, while pursuing my Bachelor of Theology (B. Th.) in Bangalore, South India, I began to feel and experience all these emotions. Just a month earlier, I had undergone a tonsillectomy. I had struggled with allergies, tonsillitis, sinusitis, and anaemia for many years before going to Bangalore for my studies. I told myself that I needed to study and become educated, so I set aside my feelings of pain and helplessness. I forced myself to attend classes even when I was very ill and did not take a break from my studies. Even when the doctor advised me to take a semester off after my tonsils were removed, I continued to study.

However, a month after my tonsillectomy, I started to go through sleeplessness, fatigue, and a feeling of complete isolation. Nobody seemed to understand my physical pain, perhaps because I hid it so well, as I did not want to be around people or talk to anybody. I cried myself to sleep practically every night. From being a very friendly, talkative person just a few months prior, I had turned into someone who only wanted to be left alone. What was I becoming?

I was experiencing depression, but I did not know it. I believed that my need to be alone was part of growing up and becoming mature. This shows how deceitful the evil thoughts were. While I felt relieved to finally acknowledge that I was physically unwell and didn't have to maintain a façade of strength in front of everyone, I was overwhelmed by a sense of helplessness. Feelings of despair often plagued my thoughts. The belief that nobody understood me made me close even more.

I did not want to share my troubled thoughts with anyone because I worried it was a sign of weakness, and I felt insecure. I was also deeply concerned about being judged as lacking spirituality and not having faith in God if I revealed any of my negative thoughts. I was under a cloud of religion rather than experiencing the freedom that Christianity offers. So, I did my best to hide any feelings of weakness or inadequacy. Even in moments when the pain and isolation fade, reflecting on those agonising years still brings back the sadness, despair, and darkness that enveloped me.

I also had many unresolved issues related to relationships within my own family. My dad and mum come from very different backgrounds, but they both belong to the same tribe. They have been married for 52 years (as of 2024), and God has helped them through many challenges and difficulties in their marriage, as well as in their lives together. However, they have not always seen things in the same light, and witnessing them disagree on almost every decision did not help my siblings and me. We were hesitant to embrace the concept of marriage and did not cultivate healthy relationships within ourselves.

My friends considered me mature, strong, thoughtful, and kind, but I was very harsh and hard on myself. I didn't know that I needed to forgive myself. You may ask, what did I need to be forgiven for? After all, it was me who was suffering. Quite simply, it was forgiveness for believing my illness was from God. Somehow, I believed God had sent the illness, not realising I was continually asking Him to heal me while all the time believing He gave it to me. I had to ask for forgiveness for my wrong thinking. My spiritual foundation had to be replaced with God's foundation.

As I have said, this is a journey of discovering ourselves in God. In that, we must adjust our thinking to His; otherwise, we will remain in the pit of illness, while the stripes that Jesus took on His back are worthless to us if we don't accept them.

> *"But He was wounded for our transgressions, He was bruised for our iniquities; The chastisement for our peace was upon Him, And **by His stripes we are healed.**"*
>
> Isaiah 53:5.

Letting Go of The Dark Night

Stuck in pain,
Much sorrow and torment,
Never knowing how to let go.
Groping about in darkness,
My soul was held captive,
My heart was writhing in pain.

The constant sting in my heart.
Of love being strangled to death in darkness.
Of my heart being shredded to pieces.
Of hope never again seeing the light of day.

The dark night of my soul continued,
existing in my body.
My heart imprisoned in a dungeon.
Bleeding and hurting,
Squeezing all life out of me.
My heart longed to be healed.

Never quite knowing how to live.
Crying in silence.
Love reached out to my heart one day.
This love was kind, forgiving,
This love is unconditional.

Love so gentle and kind.
Not judging my mistakes,
Soothing my wounds,
Ever loving, never harsh.
Only comforting.

Love that transformed my heart,
Made me live again, not just exist.
Love that made me believe again,
In the beauty of life,
Of new beginnings.

Picking up the broken pieces,
Mending the messy bits and pieces,
Another masterpiece was recreated.
My ransomed soul; now at peace.
My heart was mended and whole.
Because of Love.

This love that bore my grief.
Love that gave me beauty for ashes.
Love that replaced my regrets with hope.
This love that wiped my wounds clean.

This love is Jesus,
Lover of my soul,
Never letting me go.
My one true love,
Giving me a reason to live,
A very abundant life.

I will love you with my heart.
I will honour you with my life.
Nothing I do will make you love me any less.
My all I surrender to you wholly.

I am already cherished,
For Jesus paid the price to restore me.
Your shed blood, your broken body.
My only source of healing.

Bokali Chishi Mughavi

SECTION 1: SETTING THE STAGE

Family Dynamics and Emotional Struggles

CHAPTER 1

Early Years

"Before I formed you in the womb I knew you; Before you were born I sanctified you; I ordained you a prophet to the nations."

Jeremiah 1:5.

My parents hail from the Sumi Naga tribe (also known as the Sema tribe). Mum recounts that I was born at Naga Hospital in Kohima on February 7, 1978. She remembers every detail about when and how she went into labour and how I made my entrance into the world.

We lived in a small town named Asukhuto, also known as Khelhoshe Polytechnic Atoizu (KPA), in the Zunheboto District of Nagaland. Our town was always bustling because the polytechnic institute attracted students from all over Nagaland for their diploma programmes. Even our local Baptist church was filled with many God-fearing students on Sundays, some of whom were talented singers and musicians. Most of the teaching staff were from out of state, making Asukhuto a multi-tribal, multi-lingual town.

Asukhuto had a Government Primary School (GPS) and a privately run English medium school called King David School, which my parents started in 1985. There was a dire need for an English medium school at Khelhoshe Polytechnic Atoizu for children. The primary mode of instruction at the Government Primary School was in the Sumi dialect, which led some elders and non-local Khelhoshe Polytechnic Atoizu staff to encourage and even pressure my parents to start a school. They did so and managed it for over a decade.

My parents loved plants and trees, and they had a beautiful garden in their backyard. It looked more like a fruit orchard, with plum trees, guava plants, sugar cane, and mulberry trees. I remember our grapevine that crept upon a huge trellis, and in the summer months, we would pluck the grapes under the trellis and fill our buckets and baskets. There was also a peach tree in the front yard, which bore many fruits year after year. And how can I forget the huge cherry tree that produced cherries each year? Those berries would tempt us to eat them, and each year, my sister Agholi and I would fall to the temptation and take a bite, only to screw up our faces immediately because they were always so bitter. We would laugh at how the cherry tree tricked us each year. Other times, when no one was looking, we would climb the fruit trees and pick mulberries. These are the most beautiful memories I have of my childhood at my parents' house in Asukhuto.

To give you a breakdown of our family: I am the only biological child of my parents, but I am blessed with six more siblings, who became part of our family through adoption. I will address them by the names we call them at home.

Aqhe, the oldest sister, is a happily married woman with three beautiful kids. She is a Hindi language teacher in the city where we all now live. Strangely enough, she married a man who also hails from my dad's native village. Like my parents, she is a gifted gardener and raises her own chickens for her family's consumption which is a gift I do not possess.

Agholi is second in line. I call her Gilas because a South Indian teacher mispronounced her name, and I have continued to call her Gilas since we were seven and eight years old. Gilas is my second cousin who became my sister when I was six and she was seven. Everyone around us thinks I am older than her because she is petite and I was always the gawky, taller one. She doesn't know it, but she has beautiful eyes, great hair, and amazing skin. She is a beauty, though she doesn't realise it. Since we were just one year apart, we grew up like friends until I went away for higher studies and couldn't spend much time at home anymore. She also became a language teacher at a Government Higher Secondary School near my parents' house. She is married to a very smart math teacher Hokugha Yeptho, and they are blessed with three intelligent children.

Ruth (Rumbo) is my younger sister, a gifted and competent nurse with two nursing degrees and an MBA in healthcare. She has pretty much given up her career to be a caregiver to our aging parents. She also helps me tend to my three growing children and loves taking care of every sick person around her. Ruth loves cats just like I love plants, and though we are like chalk and cheese, I can't imagine life without her. My children love her deeply, and we feel so blessed to have Rumbo in our lives. It is not lost on us that she has had to sacrifice much to be near our parents and to take care of my children and me. Throughout my surgeries and raising kids, Ruth has been a very integral part of our lives, and I am so grateful to God for having a sister who is a great nurse yet has remained childlike in many ways. She still accompanies me on all my trips to the doctor every few months.

Bokato is next. We all call him Bokas. He became part of our family when I was 19 and has always been a very active, friendly person that everyone loves to hang out with. He is a great cook, a goofball, and a cleanliness freak. Bokas is a great uncle to our children, and the best thing about him is that he is a devout young man. He has had his struggles in relationships, but God has been faithful in his life. He started working right after high school at my husband's company and has slowly worked his way up to now taking care of various projects. We call him a multi-purpose guy because he is great with anyone he interacts with, and he is very committed to everything he does.

Viketo, whom we call Avike, is our youngest brother. He is finishing his Master's Degree in Rural Development at St. Joseph's University in our city. He is a very quiet young man, and while he has all the characteristics of the youngest in the family, he is slowly stepping up in terms of responsibilities at home. As is usual in our Naga culture, all unmarried single people live with our parents or with married siblings and share the workload. Avike is now that unmarried single young man from our family doing his bit to be there for our aging parents.

Friends and family who know us well understand that, despite our differences in appearance and manner, we are bound by a deep love forged through shared experiences over many years. These shared experiences include family jokes, relationship dramas, differences of opinion, bonding over family prayer meetings, marrying and leaving our parents' home, having children of our own, and seeing our parents' become grandparents and spoil our kids.

From the age of 5 until I was 16 years old, I suffered frequent and severe nosebleeds. The longest time I went without a nosebleed during that period was two weeks. My nose bled every month, and I vividly remember the smell and taste of fresh blood trickling into my mouth if I tried to lift my head, as the doctor advised to stop the bleeding. To this day, the sight of fresh blood makes me uncomfortable.

These nosebleeds were so frequent that I often had to return home during school hours, which was embarrassing and isolating. I felt like the odd one out, not just in my class but in the whole school. I secretly carried handkerchiefs in my school bag and the pocket of my school uniform, trying not to draw attention to myself when using them. My parents took me to several doctors who prescribed various medicines, but none provided a lasting solution.

Despite my health issues, my family's support and love helped me cope with these challenges. Our family prayer meetings and shared experiences created a strong bond that was crucial during difficult times. Reflecting on those years, I realise how much my family's unity and faith sustained me through my struggles.

As a young teenager trying to discover who I was in this world; sadly, I had to conclude that there was no cure for my nosebleeds through medications, whatever I thought, it was going to be. It caused me great sadness as I realised I was not in control of my life, but I was controlled by my nosebleeds which then caused sickness, in turn, there would be days I would be in bed, mostly because I often felt extraordinarily tired. In the summers, when my friends would come to our home and ask me to play outside, my parents' answer was always "No" because they were always worried about my weak health. It wasn't that I didn't want to play with them, but the direct heat of the sun would cause my nose to start bleeding again. As a result, I couldn't join my friends outside as much as I wanted to. By the time I was seven years old, I would get so weak from missing a meal that I would start shivering. At ten, I began having terrible headaches that would force me to bed, but even sleep didn't help. In the winter months, my joints and muscles would ache badly because of the cold weather, so I would wrap my legs with scarves to keep warm. With all this happening, I sometimes wondered if life was worth living and I was not even a teenager yet.

I was raised in a Christian family with the Bible at the centre of our beliefs. My mum made it mandatory for us to attend prayer meetings every evening. Our family altar was where we bonded over singing hymns and contemporary worship songs and took turns reading the Bible in our dialect. Besides family time, I spent a lot of time reading Bible stories and fairy tales. I came to realise that man was never going to sort out my health, only God could. One of the Bible verses that I held close to my heart was Romans 8:28: "*All things work together for good to them that love God.*"

I wonder if you were like me, sometimes questioning God. Yes, I have questioned Him. I would ask, "Did I not love God enough?", "Does God not love me?" "Why is this happening to me?" Most of the time, there was silence.

My parents were hardworking people. While they both worked full-time, they also lived in different places. My dad moved every few years to whichever town he was posted to. He served as a headmaster in government high schools and retired in 2004 as the Assistant Director of the Directorate of School Education with the Government of Nagaland, after serving in various capacities in teaching and administration for three decades.

My mum settled down with the family in Asukhuto, where she was a Government Primary School teacher. She also managed an English-medium school for over a decade. Even at the age of 73, she remains an industrious and hardworking woman though she is not as energetic as she used to be. She taught, managed, and worked in the women's department of our church for as long as we lived in that small town, always ensuring we had prayer meetings every night.

Throughout the 1980s, Mum worked with the Sumi Women's Organization (Sumi Totimi Hoho, or STH) and the women's department of our tribal Baptist association, the Sumi Baptist Akukuhou Kuqhakulu (SBAK). She also cared for many sick people in our community and helped many women give birth, despite not being a trained nurse or midwife.

Between the ages of 10 and 12, I attended two boarding schools in the towns of Kohima and Zunheboto. I hated every moment of being away from home and ran away from both schools. After I ran away for the third time in the spring of 1990, my parents decided I should stay with my dad. Consequently, I went to study in another small town, far from where my mum lived.

I was admitted to Baptist English School in Tening town, Peren District. Just as I was becoming acquainted with new friends and the lovely weather of Tening, my dad was transferred to yet another place.

I was in seventh grade, and summer was over, which meant I had to find another school. That year alone, I studied in three different schools. I didn't want to study in the new town of Medziphema, where my dad was posted. My mum found another school in Zunheboto, a hilly district of the Sumi tribe to which I belong. I attended Seven Home School in Zunheboto from August 1990 until the following year.

In early 1993, my parents decided that my mum should leave our small town and move to Dimapur because my dad was posted there again. This decision was significant because my parents had lived in Asukhuto (KPA) for about 20 years, and we were leaving behind not only our house and other properties but also many memories with neighbours, friends, and church members. At that time, finishing tenth grade was considered equivalent to finishing high school in Nagaland because the secondary school education system (eleventh and twelfth grades) was introduced much later.

Even though we lived in a small town with limited activities and outings, I was fortunate that my parents taught me the importance of reading. I was often lost in the worlds of my imagination, and my biggest dream was to live a healthy life without nosebleeds. I also dreamt about traveling around the world when I grew up.

> *"And we know that all things work together for good to those who love God, to those who are the called according to His purpose."*
>
> Romans 8:28.

CHAPTER 2

Jesus Touched Me – My First Miracle

"Then you will call upon Me and go and pray to Me, and I will listen to you."

Jeremiah 29:12.

In the spring of 1994, I believe I was given a second chance at life because of the miracle I experienced. I am still in awe of what took place. The healing I received has no other explanation than the fact that I was touched by the Lord Jesus Himself. However, before I recount the miracle, I need to share what took place before and the struggles of darkness I had to go through.

I was raised in a Baptist church by a very devout, born-again Christian mother who strongly believes in the power of prayer and divine healing. Even though I had no real faith that God could heal me from my pain and misery, I still prayed from time to time, even as a seven-year-old. I developed a strong defence against all kinds of emotional pain by shutting down my ability to feel sad or cry.

I had a different personality when I was with my friends: always jolly, never appearing serious, and constantly making everyone laugh with my jokes. However, I was a very serious and dutiful daughter. I grew up attending Sunday school regularly, which started before I went to boarding school. I led our family prayer meetings, memorised many scripture verses, and helped with all household chores whenever I came home for holidays during summer and winter breaks. Despite having changed schools seven times before I finished high school, I was able to maintain decent grades (though I was not a A-student).

In March 1994, my mother, the oldest of nine siblings, went to a prayer house with her family, far away from our small town of Asukhuto (KPA). She told me about a dream she had while at the prayer house. In her dream, she saw all kinds of worms, dirt, and insects being cleansed from my nose, and she was helping me clean up, holding me as the unclean things came out. She confidently told me I would be completely healed of my nosebleeds. I did not take her dream seriously at first. However, I went through April and May without experiencing any nosebleeds, and I realised that God had revealed my healing to my mum.

By July 1994, I enrolled in Patkai Christian College (PCC), completely healed of my nosebleeds, and began a new chapter of my life. I was blessed with wonderful roommates in both the first and second years of my pre-university (now known as Higher Secondary in India, equivalent to a High School Diploma in America and GCSE in the UK). During the first year, our dorms consisted of big rooms with five girls in each room. In the second year, some of us were moved to a bigger building where three girls shared a room. I preferred this new building because it had a more conducive environment and fewer people to deal with in a room.

Life as a college student at 16 was fun because I was more social and made many friends without having to worry about my nosebleeds, which God had healed me from. My friends and I were always chatting, joking, teasing each other, imitating our lecturers, and eating a lot of junk food. Every Saturday evening, a group of us would dress up and attend the Evangelical Union (EU) services at the College Chapel.

For the first time in my young life, I was healthy and genuinely happy without having to pretend. However, there were nights when I felt alone and confused about where my life was headed. Those two years at Patkai were life-changing for me, especially when I started attending EU (Evangelical Union) services every Saturday and heard great testimonies from guest speakers, student leaders, and lecturers. I began to understand the importance of having a personal relationship with Jesus Christ.

Even though I had always prayed, fasted, and believed strongly in the power of prayer, I had not truly committed to making Jesus Christ my Lord and personal Saviour. During my two-year studies at PCC, a preacher from Mizoram named Rev. Van Lal Ngakha visited and delivered a sermon at our EU service. His simple yet deeply moving presentation of the gospel resonated profoundly with me. For the first time in my life, I understood that Jesus had already paid the price for my salvation and that my eternity was secured if I was willing to commit my life to a living relationship with Him. I began to grasp that the Son of God had given up the splendours of heaven to come to this world, to die and save me from my sins. I felt liberated knowing that the Creator of this world loved me deeply.

However, even though I had accepted Jesus Christ as my Lord and personal Saviour and was willing to follow and serve Him, I continued to live with the idea that I could somehow please God with my good works, believing that I could earn His love and blessings by being very hard on myself. I never quite understood the message of God's grace. By the time I was in the second year of Pre-University, I had slowly begun to yield to the voice in my heart, suggesting that I should pursue theological studies and learn more about God. I was perhaps the most zealous girl, eager to learn more about God and open to everything that Bible college had to offer.

In the summer of 1997, a few months after I finished my pre-university exams, I joined New Life College (NLC) in the South Indian city of Bangalore. I began the application process a few months before my final exams at PCC and was soon accepted to do a Bachelor of Theology programme at NLC.

"For by grace you have been saved through faith, and that not of yourselves; it is the gift of God."

Ephesians 2:8.

CHAPTER 3

Loneliness and Despair

"And He said to me, My grace is sufficient for you, for My strength is made perfect in weakness. Therefore most gladly I will rather boast in my infirmities, that the power of Christ may rest upon me."

2 Corinthians 12:9.

Life in Bible college was quite different from what I had expected. I had imagined it to be spirit-filled, with perfect people who were like angels. My unrealistic expectations, ignorance, and limited understanding of Bible college students makes me cringe when I think about it now. To my great shock and horror, Bible college was filled with imperfect and insecure people just like me. To say I was disappointed would be an understatement. In the first year, I kept thinking that Bible college wasn't for someone like me, even though I enjoyed studying most of the subjects and disciplines offered at NLC.

Despite the many disappointments, I was happy to be introduced to all the foundational courses of the Old Testament and the New Testament, theological concepts, basic psychology, attending chapel, hearing inspiring guest speakers, and so on. My toughest challenge was living under one roof in the dormitory with so many imperfect people. Reflecting on myself now, I feel a sense of embarrassment, realising how judgmental I was towards every other student, consumed by self-righteousness. Every little weakness I saw in a person at the dormitory, classroom, or college bothered and angered me. I was also very vocal in condemning people whom I thought did not live up to the standards of a good Bible college student. I was miserable as I made everyone around me uncomfortable, even though some girlfriends seemed to like the fact that I could sing, lead in worship, and consistently maintain very good grades until my second year.

God, in His great mercy, helped me confront my own weaknesses, judgmental attitude, and self-righteousness through the classroom teachings and explorations of the Bible by our lecturers, witnessing faithful servant leaders among the faculty members, and experiencing love and grace from some senior friends who had gone through similar transformations. The process of transformation was long, hard, and painful. God always reached out to me in ways that made me realise and understand the depth of His love for me—mostly through reading the Word, but also through sermons and testimonies of our lecturers and guest speakers, and many times, through deliverance amid difficult circumstances.

One day, during my second year, I was too ill to attend classes and stayed back at the dorm on sick leave. Feeling very lonely and despondent, I cried and prayed for a long time, seeking God's intervention in my life. I was tired of feeling helpless and powerless about my recurring physical ailments. After praying, I opened my Bible randomly and found myself in Romans Chapter 5. To my utter surprise and joy, every word and sentence in those verses spoke directly to my heart and brought me great comfort.

My struggles with self-righteousness, my desire to always be the best but never living up to my own standards, my inability to accept my failures, my inability to surrender completely to Jesus despite having made the commitment to do so, and my health issues resurfacing despite being healed from nosebleeds—all weighed heavily on me. However, after reading a portion of scripture in the Book of Romans, I felt so light, understood, and loved by a saviour as personal as Jesus Christ. Let me share them with you:

> *"And not only that, but we also glory in tribulations, knowing that tribulation produces perseverance; and perseverance, character; and character, hope. Now hope does not disappoint, because the love of God has been poured out in our hearts by the Holy Spirit who was given to us."*
>
> Romans 5:3-5.

I remain extremely grateful to the Holy Spirit for ministering to me that day in a very personal way.

I consistently maintained good grades during the first two years of my bachelor studies at NLC. However, towards the end of the second year, my grades dropped because I began to experience deep sadness and wanted to be left alone most of the time. I, who used to be the life of every gathering, started feeling very uncomfortable around people. I did not know what was happening to me. I became inconsistent in everything I did. I began to despise being around people. I could not concentrate on my studies or stay focused as I had during the first two years. I was very unhappy during my final year at NLC because I did not know who I was anymore, nor did I understand why I felt so badly about myself all the time. I treated myself very poorly.

A part of me wanted to remain the happy-go-lucky girl I used to be, but many parts of me had changed. I felt increasingly sad and could not pinpoint the reason for my sadness. I felt the world closing in on me. Never had I felt so alone. I felt no one understood my darkness, so I did not try to explain to anyone why I was sad. Everyone around me noticed and commented that I had changed so much. Yet, I thought that being unhappy and sad was part of growing up. From 1997 to

1999, I had very few moments of laughter, and I still wonder how I was able to fake being normal for so long. It drained the life out of me, distorted my thought process, and turned me into someone I didn't want to be—a negative, scared, angry, wounded, and confused woman.

By the time I finished my degree, I had only managed to graduate with a few 'B's. I blamed and hated myself even more because I had convinced myself that I wasn't, and would never be, good enough without good grades. Even as I write this now, I shudder because I realise how mentally and emotionally unstable I was at that time. I did not know I needed to seek help. I was losing my focus, nothing excited me, and all I wanted was to disappear from the face of the earth. I had no inkling that the mental illness, which ran on my mother's side of the family, was beginning to surface in my life.

Looking back now, I truly wish I had someone to share my struggles with back then. I wish someone had told me that there was more to life than just making straight 'A's. I was so fixated on how useless I felt without good grades that my value and worth as a person were completely dependent on my performance in front of others, including my parents and extended family. The need to please my parents and my family weighed heavily on my shoulders as a child, and I took it upon myself to make everyone proud of me—even if it meant killing myself emotionally.

I graduated from New Life College with a Bachelor of Theology Degree in February 1999 and went back to Nagaland. I carried with me a load of memories—some funny, many painful and transformative— but also wounds that I still did not know how to deal with. Little did I know that the years ahead would be extremely dark, quite scary, and even more painful.

> *"Come to Me, all you who labor and are heavy laden, and I will give you rest."*
>
> Matthew 11:28.

CHAPTER 4

Darkness of the Soul

"The LORD is near to those who have a broken heart,
And saves such as have a contrite spirit."

Psalm 34:18.

A couple of months after my graduation, while I was at home, I had my first emotional breakdown. I was still nursing a wound that I couldn't let go of, and it was eating me up. Back in the summer of 1997, when I had my tonsils removed, two older friends had gone out of their way to take care of me after my parents, who had come to be with me in Bangalore, had to leave after three weeks. While I was very grateful to have older friends who wanted to protect and care for me physically, I began to feel very controlled by them, especially by an older female friend I had taken to be my foster sister. I did not realise it back then, but many years later, I understood that differences in upbringing and value systems can affect the way we relate to others.

I make friends easily and enjoy getting to know people. There were a few out-of-college events at other churches where we would go for choir practices with other church members, including workshops and seminars we had to attend. However, I felt judged whenever this sister started spreading lies about me, and I felt my character was being constantly assassinated. I was labelled a spoiled kid, which hurt me deeply. To this day, I still do not know why she felt so threatened by me. She was already in her early 30s, and I was a 19-year-old who looked up to her and trusted her. I also cared deeply about her and often helped her with her assignments because she needed assistance.

I bottled up my feelings and started to feel numb and lifeless. Our relationship soured to the point where I stopped talking to her completely. I wrote her a letter stating that I would never be able to trust her again. She apologised, but it could not undo the immense pain she had caused a struggling 19-year-old girl. I also did not know how to let go of that pain because I had no one ministering to me, nor did I know of anyone who could help me. It was after a decade that I was able to slowly let go of the pain of this particular experience.

In the spring of 1999, I experienced my first-ever emotional breakdown. My parents were facing significant difficulties because my father was unjustly demoted and transferred after a junior staff member falsely accused him of an offence he did not commit. This event hurt my dad very deeply, and I questioned God as to why the corrupt thrive while the honest ones have to suffer. My parents' spiritual quests were also on different levels. Even though my parents had a very traditional marriage, my siblings and I experienced no lasting peace at home. They never seemed to agree on anything, which made my siblings and I very anxious most of the time. My dad seemed miserable, especially after being demoted and transferred to a place he did not like at all, while my mum was hanging on to life only because of her faith in Christ. I had grown up witnessing my mum's brokenness, and it was painful to see her still struggling to keep everything together.

Anxiety was a major part of my life by then, and although I had managed to hide it from others until I graduated, it was very clear by April and May that I was losing the battle to keep myself together. I don't remember if it was April or May, but during those months, I struggled to sleep, cried day and night, couldn't eat, and couldn't function normally. My poor mother didn't know what to do with me. While she was there for me, encouraging me to think positively, I felt judged and condemned because I was constantly reminded by Mom that I had no faith in God, that I was not strong, and so on. I felt I had failed my mother, who had raised me to be a strong woman of God, which made me very angry and disappointed in myself. I had failed to make her proud by not getting the best grades in the final year of my bachelor's degree. Now, I had failed her even more by losing control of my emotions.

I hated feeling so miserable and out of control. I, who had always encouraged my parents and friends to be strong and positive, had completely lost my drive and my ability to dream and pursue that dream. Most of all, I felt life was not even worth living. All I wanted was to die, but I knew that taking my own life was out of the question because I knew how much it would hurt my parents to lose me. Even in my broken state, I knew that my parents loved me very much—had it not been for their love, I would have taken my own life because the thought of dying was much more appealing to me than living with so much pain day in and day out. I felt I was a burden and a disgrace to my family. Although my family loved me and never made me feel like a burden, those thoughts arose from my helpless feelings growing up, being sick and often dependent on my loved ones to take care of me. I hated the feeling of being so dependent, lying in bed, and being taken to doctors and hospitals every now and then. I had no idea how much pain and ugly feelings I had suppressed, which were now resurfacing, making me feel out of control and extremely helpless.

My mother did the only thing she knew best. She took me to a prayer house, now known as Ayinato Healing and Prayer Centre, about a 45-minute drive away from Dimapur city, where we had been residing for the past five years. She fasted and prayed with me for five days. It was a quiet place, so I had enough time to talk to my mum about the things that were disturbing me. I did not understand it back then, but because Mum had gone through and survived so many heartaches and difficult experiences and had come out stronger in her faith, she seemed to constantly remind me of how weak my own faith was. It was not a good feeling to be reminded every now and then that I did not have faith in God, although I knew she meant well. I was 21 years old by then, and I felt very old but also did not know that my emotional and mental breakdown had happened because it had been building up for many years due to the various types of traumas and physical pain I had endured throughout my childhood until my breakdown.

By the end of the five-day fast, I regretted that I had lost my ability to keep it together. I felt guilty for feeling sad and tired of my life, and I believed that I had committed a great sin by feeling hopeless. By the end of the fast, I was determined never to make the same mistake of taking my life for granted or feeling sad and worried. The problem, though, was that what I needed at that time was rest, long-term counselling, and not just a five-day fast.

I realised many years later, during therapy in 2007, that it wasn't my fault to have felt so completely broken. The anxiety, anger, fear, doubts, and helplessness had been building up ever since I was a little girl. I was and am human enough to have valid reasons to feel helpless, desperate, and even confused and angry at the injustice my family and I had suffered on so many levels.

I didn't know any better, and I wish someone had told me that it wasn't my fault that I was experiencing a breakdown, that others also go through this, and that even prophets and psalmists in the Bible went through breakdowns and depressive episodes.

The five-day fast helped me regain some perspective about my darkness of mind and soul, but my ability to suppress all my dark feelings—anger at myself and others, anger towards God for the pain and shame of my mother's family—did not last long. The dark, unresolved anger and pain kept resurfacing in my life for many more years to come.

There was nobody I could turn to apart from my mother because I had grown up being very protected. I had always been a good girl in school, a good student at Bible college, constantly cheering others up and encouraging everyone. I had no one to talk to or share my dark emotional experiences with. As far as I was concerned, if my mum, who had gone through so much pain in life, was still a survivor, I had no reason for my emotional breakdown to be validated. Little did I know that I was headed towards another decade of a lonely and dark journey that would include breakdowns, an inability to function, and feeling completely hopeless to the point of being suicidal.

In 1999, I was accepted at the Oriental Theological Seminary (OTS) in Nagaland for a Master of Divinity programme. My junior year at OTS went by quickly. I often cried myself to sleep every night during my first semester. Even so, nobody would have believed that I was so lonely, scared, confused, angry, or worried. We were two girls who made it to the M.Div. programme that academic year, but the other girl dropped out shortly after school started, leaving me as the only girl in my academic year. While I had girlfriends in the dorm, my classmates were all boys/young men. They were all very kind to me and treated me like their sister, and I did my best to reciprocate their kindness, but it felt strange and lonely not to have girls in the classroom. After a few classes, we had a sister from the Master of Ministry (M. Min) programme join us, which added to the number of girls in the classroom. However, while I have always been a friendly person and had no problems adapting to new environments (or so I had convinced myself), I began to find that I liked being by myself again. At first, I thought that was a good thing, but I soon began to despise being around people. I wanted to study by myself, do my assignments by myself, and lock myself up in my room when there were no community gatherings.

The good thing about being at OTS at that time was the emphasis on building a beloved community by the faculty and staff. Apart from training students to pursue academic excellence, we were expected to participate in community programmes, including sports. Attending the mandatory Friday football matches was torturous for me, even though I faked my way through it all very well, pretending that I enjoyed attending and cheering during the matches. During most days in my first year, I was on hormonal medication and spent sleepless nights reading and writing assignments—which, of course, did not help my drowsiness during the day. Because I faked my behaviour so well, I was already gaining the reputation of being a 'tough girl'. The Principal called me a 'tough cookie' in his Colloquium on Personality Development (which was not graded but was a pass/fail mandatory course).

The first year went by quickly; the next two years seemed like an eternity to me. Back then, OTS had three academic quarters per year, and it was challenging to manage community life, spiritual activities, weekend practical ministries in the surrounding villages, and academic rigour. I did not want to admit for a year that I still carried so much sadness in my heart. I did not know how to let go and had nobody to encourage me to let go of so many painful memories and experiences. It made me sadder by the day. I was an expert in encouraging others but had no idea how to seek help. The only person I could open up to was my friend Ellen, who is now a reputed psychotherapist. She helped me cope during my first year by taking time to talk to me and encourage me by writing notes and reading the scriptures to me when we were both less busy. However, she was two years ahead of me, so she graduated exactly a year after I joined the seminary.

In the spring of 2001, during my second year at OTS, I experienced another complete emotional breakdown. Just as in the past when I had experienced terrible feelings of isolation, deep sadness, and helplessness, this time around, I felt alone, even though I was living in a small community of close-knit lecturers, professors, and fellow students who genuinely cared for me. I skipped an exam because of my breakdown, and a very kind lecturer wrote me a long letter of encouragement, for which I have always been grateful. My body, mind, spirit, and soul were all screaming for rest. I was so tired of life. All I wanted to do was sleep and never wake up. I did not want to eat. I could not sleep at night. All

I felt was anger at myself. I was very tired throughout the day and in pain, both physically and emotionally, at night.

Everyone noticed my quietness and lethargy towards everything, which made it even worse. I called my mum from a landline phone that students were allowed to use and asked her to come and take me home because I wanted to take a break from my studies for a semester. Sadly, my mother did not understand why I wanted to take a break, and she told me there was no way she was going to allow me to give up on my studies. This added to my feeling of extreme helplessness. I will never forget how rejected and helpless I felt that day walking back to my dorm after the phone call.

If my own mother could not understand my need to take a break, there was no way anyone else would ever understand me. Even as I recollect the incident and the day I made the call to my mother, I still grieve for the girl who felt so trapped in her own mind, her spirit tortured and her soul tormented, with no one understanding her.

Since I had practically no one who understood me, or at least that is how I felt, I went about like a zombie, attending classes every day but never really being able to concentrate on anything, going back to my room and crying myself to sleep most nights. This was my situation from the spring of 2001 until I graduated in the summer of 2002. Everything seemed to drag on. I have no words to describe the torment I felt until the day I graduated from OTS.

During the three years of my M.Div. studies, I was diagnosed with typhoid four times and had to go home for medical treatment three times in one school year alone. During my first year, I had also been on medication for six months for hormonal imbalance. I had grown up skinny and unhealthy due to my many health issues. I lost so much weight that by the end of my M.Div. programme, I weighed 46 kgs (101 lbs). I looked like a walking skeleton wrapped in skin. My heart always ached, my mind was always disturbed, and my soul felt trapped and wounded. I was full of shame, anger, confusion, and helplessness, all at the same time. The worst part was that I did not know how to stop feeling like that. I felt like a ghost, not a person. God blessed me with genuine friends who cared for me, but I could not bring myself to believe that I was worthy of receiving anyone's love and care. I believed all the lies of the enemy of my soul, that I was indeed worthless, and that nobody would ever truly understand how I felt.

Deep down in my heart was a throbbing pain. I was not able to give my best to my studies because of the darkness that I felt all the time. Despite my health issues, I had been a fairly good student. I cruised through high school and Pre-University years without studying much and got very decent grades. However, when I decided to pursue theological studies, I began to study very hard and committed myself to academic excellence. I had every intention of pursuing higher studies and being involved in the teaching profession. While doing my first degree, I wanted to pursue counselling but began to develop a love for church history while doing my M.Div.

Dr. Joshua Lorin, who is now the Principal of OTS, was the lecturer for Historical Theology back when I was a junior in my M.Div. course. Even though he taught us for only a year, I was fascinated by how he taught us the history of the early church through to the age of modern church history, with so much passion and vigour. His detailed explanations and descriptions of the Reformation era really struck a chord with me. I loved reading about John Calvin, Martin Luther, and other reformers of the church in my first year.

In the meantime, I tried very hard to be confident and believe in myself. However, year after year, I crumbled inside. I tried hard to convince myself that I was fine. I began to realise that my memory was not as good as it had been earlier. I had attended a few boarding schools and had learned to adapt to new environments, make new friends, and stayed in touch with most of my old friends, even in the era of snail mail and landlines. After I began to experience the darkness of my mind and thoughts, I stopped staying in touch with my old friends, some of whom were my childhood friends. I began to lose many parts of myself without even realising I was losing them.

I also ended up feeling even more confused about where my life was headed and what I truly wanted to do. By the middle of 2002, I had graduated from Oriental Theological Seminary. I was ashamed that I did not graduate with the grades I wanted to achieve, although I did not do too badly. The obsessive feeling of not being able to live up to my own expectations made me very angry with myself. All I felt was self-loathing.

Looking back now, I wish I had been kind to myself, but I could never rest in the thought that it is okay not to be perfect at all times and in all ways. I confided in only two friends, who told me a few times that I should stop living in the past. I did not realise it then, but years later, when I sought therapy, I understood that I had relived many memories from 1997 over and over again, rehashing the pain I suffered physically and emotionally, being far away from my parents, the feeling of isolation, and being dependent on others after my tonsillectomy. Although the removal of tonsils is considered to be a very minor surgery in most countries, mine was different because I had a very painful inflammation of the tonsils, which made it difficult for me to even breathe, and I had to be on medication for two weeks before I had them removed. My parents had come down to Bangalore, where I was studying then, and had been with me throughout the surgery and post-surgery as well. They left after three weeks because of my adamant decision not to take a break from my studies. My mum kept on asking me to take a semester's break and allow my body some rest, all to no avail. Not long after my surgery, my feelings of despair started, although I had no clue as to why I was feeling that way.

During that period, I saw my parents go through some difficulties, and it troubled me that I could not help them. I saw my dad suffer injustice from people he knew very well and had been close to at some point in time. I felt helpless seeing my dad suffer not because he was dishonest but because he held on to his Christian values and maintained his integrity to the end. God is faithful and has proven His goodness to our family over the years in many ways, but at that time, I could not make sense of how a very honest man was made to suffer for no fault of his. The whole family was affected. It was hard to watch my dad suffer disappointment after disappointment for years with regard to his job, serving the government of Nagaland, where I witnessed corruption of the highest order first-hand. Many times, my dad was a pawn at the hands of bureaucrats and politicians. I do not in any way want to condemn or pinpoint anyone personally because God has proven Himself faithful to my parents for standing up to ungodliness. However, I can testify that even today we have many church going Naga bureaucrats and politicians who do not represent God's justice, nor do they care about treating honest people with the dignity and respect they deserve. Love of power and money abound both in government and in the society.

During my struggle with depression, I kept a journal of all my emotional and mental experiences. However, I was scared that others would read my journals and come to know of my self-loathing, negativity, fears, anger, and all the dark emotions I felt. So, at the end of the year, I would tear them up and burn all my diaries and journals. This habit continued for almost 10 years.

The only thing that kept me going was my spiritual upbringing. My mother had taught me about the importance of prayer and reading the Bible. So, while my feelings of hopelessness were real and suicide was often on my mind, I resorted to prayer most times.

In 2018, the NGO I am associated with conducted a workshop on Mental Health and Wellness and invited Dr. Ellen Jamir (nee Konyak) as a resource person. She started her session by reading Psalm 88. Every verse from this Psalm made me realise that the Psalmist had gone through the pit of darkness. The Psalmist had been slain, alienated, and abandoned as he described his feelings of helplessness.

¹ Lord, you are the God who saves me; day and night I cry out to you. ² May my prayer come before you; turn your ear to my cry. ³ I am overwhelmed with troubles and my life draws near to death. ⁴ I am counted among those who go down to the pit; I am like one without strength. ⁵ I am set apart with the dead, like the slain who lie in the grave, whom you remember no more, who are cut off from your care. ⁶ You have put me in the lowest pit, in the darkest depths. ⁷ Your wrath lies heavily on me; you have overwhelmed me with all your waves. ⁸ You have taken from me my closest friends and have made me repulsive to them. I am confined and cannot escape; ⁹ my eyes are dim with grief. I call to you, Lord, every day; I spread out my hands to you. ¹⁰ Do you show your wonders to the dead? Do their spirits rise up and praise you? ¹¹ Is your love declared in the grave, your faithfulness in Destruction? ¹² Are your wonders known in the place of darkness, or your righteous deeds in the land of oblivion? ¹³ But I cry to you for help, Lord; in the morning my prayer comes before you. ¹⁴ Why, Lord, do you reject me and hide your face from me? ¹⁵ From my youth I have suffered and been close to death; I have borne your terrors and am in despair. ¹⁶ Your wrath has swept over me; your terrors have destroyed me. ¹⁷ All day long they surround me like a flood; they have completely engulfed me. ¹⁸ You have taken from me friend and neighbour— darkness is my closest friend.

SECTION 2: TURNING POINTS

Breakthrough Experiences Equals New Horizons

CHAPTER 5

Denmark and Thailand

"Have I not commanded you? Be strong and of good courage; do not be afraid, nor be dismayed, for the LORD your God is with you wherever you go."

Joshua 1:9.

Amid all the suffering I went through during my three years of pursuing my M.Div. programme, I got a chance to travel to Denmark and Thailand, which allowed me to broaden my horizons, make new friends, and create some beautiful memories that I could hold on to in my darkest times.

During the early spring of 2000, as we were nearing the end of our junior year, six students from the junior and middle classes at OTS (three from each class) were called to the Principal's office and informed that we had been selected for a tour to Denmark during the summer break. Our trip would be funded by the Danish Baptist Union, and we would also be attending their Annual Mission Conference. We were to perform original compositions about the struggles of the Naga people by Dr. Wati Aier, the Principal of OTS at that time.

The six of us often met after class hours and on weekends to practise our traditional songs and dances, along with the songs written and arranged by our Principal. Finally, the summer break arrived, and we were all ready to travel to Denmark in July. We travelled as a group of ten people, and the trip turned out to be much more fun than I had originally anticipated. Rev. Zhabu Therhuja was the General Secretary of the Nagaland Baptist Church Council (NBCC), the late Rev. Dr. Chen Rengma was the Youth Secretary of NBCC, Dr. Zelhou Keyho was the Academic Dean of OTS, and Mr. Savi Legisie was the Board Chairman of OTS. Together with them, our travel entourage made quite a team.

For us students, this was our first trip overseas, and it was filled with many funny incidents. We played pranks on each other and took photographs of those who were tired and napping with mouths wide open in the car while travelling. We felt a sense of wonder and amazement at doors and gates being opened by remote controls and experienced the stinging cold in mid-summer at Moscow International airport during our transit. We had fun picking strawberries, as summer turned out to be strawberry picking season in Denmark, and we met many new people. We travelled from Dimapur to Kolkata, Kolkata to Moscow, and Moscow to Copenhagen, which was a long and tiring trip. I had just finished my medications for hormonal imbalance, but my general health and immune system were still not strong enough, so I experienced air sickness during our travel from Kolkata to Moscow, via Delhi.

I was so tired that I didn't realise when we reached Copenhagen. Despite the jet lag and exhaustion, I could sense the cleanliness and freshness of Denmark at the airport. A group of Danish Baptist officials picked us up at the airport and took us to Roskilde, a city next to Copenhagen. During the ride, I felt I had been transported to a land of fairy tales. Everything looked so sleek, so clean, and so soothing to my eyes. The buildings and streets appeared modern yet had an old-world charm, much like what I had seen in movies, paintings, or books.

I had grown up reading fairy tales, and the one that I really loved was *The Little Match Girl*, set in Copenhagen. I often told my sister that when I grew up, I would visit Denmark. Never in my wildest dreams did I imagine that I would actually visit Denmark and that it would be my first international trip. Back then, I thought it was a coincidence, but over the past two decades of my walk with Jesus, I have come to realise and believe that God is indeed a very personal God and that He is able to make our dreams come true, even a little girl's dream of visiting a land she had read about in fairy tales.

The few weeks in Denmark were filled with trips to churches, attending a week-long Baptist Scouts Camp at a beautiful retreat centre owned by the Danish Baptist Union, and meeting and making many new friends (a few of whom I stayed in touch with for many years and one I still keep in touch with). The highlight of the trip was attending the DBU's Missions Conference, where we met many Danish missionaries who had come from all parts of the world. Two missionary couples made a significant impression on me. One was an elderly couple who had served in Burundi, Africa, as missionaries for most of their adult life and were now retired. The other couple was a Danish medical missionary and his Bangladeshi wife, who were preparing to go to another country as medical missionaries after having served in Bangladesh. I also met a brother from Rwanda who had survived the Rwandan Genocide of 1994.

Our itinerary was packed with events, and many Danish people we met joked that even they had not visited as many Danish towns and cities as we were going to. We visited a third-generation Danish family of farmers from a Baptist church that hosted us. They showed us around their expansive rice fields and a pig farm with an uncountable number of pigs in a very clean and sanitised environment. On our third day there, we realised that potatoes were a major food item in Danish homes, so we all decided to learn the Danish word for potato—'*kartoffel*'.

I was pleasantly surprised to learn that the popular Danish band,

Michael Learns to Rock (MLTR), which I had listened to during my high school and early college years, was having a concert in Roskilde, the first city we visited in Denmark. Even though I have not been able to visit Denmark again, I still remember the lovely Danish towns, cities, ports, beaches, and countryside that we toured. So many Baptist families hosted us with love, kindness, and hospitality that, to this day, I remember my visit to Denmark as the best trip I have ever taken in my life.

There was a family that hosted us for about four days and nights in a small town during the latter part of our tour. After we left Denmark, I kept in touch with them through snail mail at first and later via emails. The family later sent me a gift of a few hundred dollars when I first went to South Korea to study. I know that their generosity towards me has been seen by God, and I will forever remain grateful to God and to them. By the time we returned home in August, my eyes had been opened, my worldview had broadened, and my horizons had definitely expanded. Visiting a Scandinavian country, seeing the sun set so late, meeting the very good-looking Nordic people from Denmark, Sweden and Norway, and seeing the very clean country of Denmark—all seemed like good medicine for my depression, which I still battled with when I was alone.

September 2000 arrived, and it was time for us to start our autumn quarter. I went back to OTS as a middler and was still the only girl in my class. The summer went by quickly with the trip to Denmark, and the rest of the summer break was spent visiting Baptist churches around Dimapur with the team, giving our testimonies, relating experiences about our trip, and completing assignments that were due. My biggest assignment was on the Canonization of the New Testament, which I had to present in front of the whole OTS community as soon as school reopened. Just as we remember the taste of a good meal, the memory of my trip to Denmark stayed with me throughout the autumn quarter until the winter break when depression began to rear its ugly head again. I did not recognise the symptoms back then and was very good at convincing myself that nothing was wrong with me, that I had left my history of breakdowns behind. The only problem I thought I had was that I was not good enough for anything, that I was worthless, incapable, and useless. I felt like the greatest phoney in the world because I really hated doing anything, but I had to survive by doing them.

I also allowed some friends to treat me as though I was of no importance, which hurt me even more. I did not know how to stop treating myself poorly and start treating myself right. Every time I faced any interpersonal relationship problems, whether with friends or family, all I wanted was to run far away from people who did not see things my way. In theory, I was learning about the concept of 'agree to disagree', a very common phrase used by our professors and lecturers at the seminary. In reality, I did not know how to disagree, and I certainly did not know how to protect or defend myself. All I did was clam up and let everyone misunderstand me, which only added to my heartache. The few people who understood me knew I had anger issues, yet I did not know how to process or express my anger in a mature way when I was being misunderstood so I would just shut them out or push them away.

Every time I heard an unkind word about me or gossip that was contrary to who I was, I did not know how to let go or clarify the issue to those making assumptions about me. Many times, I would blame myself, literally telling myself that I deserved to stay in pain. I did not feel even a tiny bit of hope that there would come a time when I would feel understood. That was why I always felt so alone and isolated, even though I was always surrounded by people.

The winter of 2000 went by quickly. Even though I had a terrible breakdown in the spring of 2001, we had another trip to look forward to in the summer. This time, the group was much bigger, and we prepared many cultural items and songs to perform, as we were set to tour many parts of Thailand. My mood swings, sadness, and anger at myself were increasing. I would be laughing and acting normal in front of friends, then go to the restroom and cry my heart out. My mind was always plagued with thoughts of how everyone thought the worst of me. In July 2001, we went from Dimapur to Kolkata and then to Bangkok, the very vibrant capital of Thailand.

Travelling from one very hot country to another very warm country in midsummer made it a trip to remember!

When we landed in Bangkok, we were questioned for over an hour at immigration. As we don't typically look like Indians, we were accused of travelling on fake passports. It was not a funny experience at the time, but I laugh about it now because whenever I travel to other countries, I often have to explain to people about the location of Nagaland on the map of India, our ethnicity, our culture, dialects, and our history with the British and now with India. However, it is never a pleasant experience to be questioned about our identity and prove our authenticity all the time.

After spending a couple of nights in Bangkok and visiting a church or two, we headed north to Chiang Mai and a Karen village named Musuki. We then travelled to Chiang Rai and more villages, mostly visiting schools run by the Church of Christ Thailand (CCT). A few alumni of OTS were teaching in those schools. Our most memorable visit was to Mae Sot on the northernmost border of Myanmar and Thailand. In the mountains bordering these two countries are many camps of Karen people, whom the Thai government has allowed to settle as Internally Displaced People, though they are not granted refugee status.

I will never be able to express in words the helplessness and despair I felt while visiting the camps. We visited a school and a college set up at Mae La Camp by the Asian Baptist Federation to help educate Karen children and the youth. Since they were not granted refugee status, they are not allowed to leave their camps in the mountains to seek jobs or further education. The living conditions of the Karen people were difficult to witness. Yet, we were welcomed with so much warmth and hospitality. To this day, I remember the delicious meals we had at the camp, the papaya salad recipe that I brought home with me, and the traditional waistcoats they gifted us. The Karen people reminded me that love and generosity are possible even with limited material resources. They welcomed us with so much love, fed us well, and even gave us gifts, despite their situation as a People group that does not even have the right to be granted refugee status.

We were also very proud of our Naga graduates of OTS, who were living at the camp and teaching the youth, despite not having many facilities. Their commitment to serving God's people, who are forsaken by the world, is a pleasing sacrifice unto the Lord. I am honoured to call two of them my friends—Dr. Sashi Jamir and Rev. Dr. Ellen Konyak Jamir. They are now married, have two beautiful daughters, and continue to serve God and His Kingdom through teaching and various ministries.

We concluded our visit to northern Thailand by visiting the Golden Triangle, where Myanmar, Thailand, and Laos meet. We then returned to Bangkok, did some shopping, and after three weeks of travelling to countless towns, villages, and a few cities in Thailand, we headed back home to Nagaland. During this time, I was losing weight, and the pain of unexplainable sadness and deep loneliness kept increasing. On the outside, I managed to act normal, but I knew something was very wrong with me. Inside, I was screaming with pain, feeling trapped and helpless.

By the first week of September, we were back at the seminary. It felt strange to be a senior and even stranger to be in a class where I was the only female who would be graduating the next year. I was able to take my comprehensive exams, both written and oral, and thankfully, I finished them without panic attacks. Our principal, who taught us Systematic Theology, spoke words of encouragement to me when he noticed how nervous I was during my oral defence of my paper on the Resurrection.

The academic session started in September 2001, and I managed my senior year of the M.Div. programme without another emotional breakdown. However, the year did not go by without feelings of being trapped and helpless in my darkness. I still cried many nights and felt very angry at myself for feeling so weak and tired of life.

Looking back today, I feel so grateful that I was able to finish my M.Div. Degree without giving up. During the Convocation, the Academic Dean, Dr. Zelhou Keyho, described me as a very strong girl. I have often wondered what he would have said if he had known how broken, fragmented, and tormented I had felt all those years as his student.

> *"The LORD will give strength to His people;*
> *The LORD will bless His people with peace."*
>
> Psalm 29:11.

CHAPTER 6

Dreams and Revelations

"Trust in the LORD with all your heart, and lean not on your own understanding."

Proverbs 3:5.

By the summer of 2002, I was ready for a change of scenery. A month and a half after completing my M.Div. Degree, I travelled to Bangalore to teach at the same college where I had done my B.Th. During my senior year at OTS, we would often pray at our weekly prayer meetings for students who were about to graduate. I also prayed very sincerely many times, wondering what the Lord wanted me to do after graduation. I had no clue where I was heading. Every time I prayed about my future and slept, I dreamed I was back at my alma mater, NLC.

Strangely enough, two months before my graduation, while at home one weekend, I received a telegram from Mrs. Mary Thannickal, wife of the founder and principal of New Life College, Dr. Thannickal. The telegram read: 'Come back to NLC, God will open doors.' I was pleasantly surprised to be asked to teach at my alma mater, but I was also quickly reminded of the dreams I had the past year about being back at NLC.

My mother did not agree with or support the idea of going back to teach at my old college; she said it would do me no good and strongly believed it was not God's will. Strangely enough, for the first time in my life, my dad supported me and thought it would be a good thing for me to go back and teach at NLC. In the past, my dad had always held me back from going anywhere outside of Nagaland because of my health issues. This time, however, my mum was very adamant, so I asked her to pray and see if God would speak to her because I was convinced that it was God leading me to Bangalore again. A month after we received the telegram, my mum attended a prayer-and-fast meeting with some of her friends. She was praying about what I should do after my graduation because another Bible college in Nagaland was also asking me to come and teach. I knew she wanted me to stay near home, not far away. When I came home for a weekend a few weeks before my graduation, my mum told me she was convinced it was God's will for me to go and teach at NLC in Bangalore. Even though I was not surprised by her change of mind, I was curious about how God had spoken to her to convince her about His leading me to Bangalore.

My mother explained that, during the prayer and fast, a song kept coming to her mind. The original song is in our dialect, and the literal translation goes something like this:

> *I will sing for Jesus.*
> *Wherever in the world I go,*
> *Whether I cross rivers or lands,*
> *I will sing for Jesus.*

> *I must preach about Jesus.*
> *Wherever in the world I go,*
> *Whether I cross rivers or lands,*
> *I must preach about Jesus.*

My mum told me that the Holy Spirit reminded her of the many times she had prayed over me in my younger years, dedicating my life to God and His service, especially during the years when my nosebleeds had been very severe and leading up to God healing me. She was reminded that God would take care of me wherever He led me and that she was convicted of her lack of belief in God's plans and direction for my life. I must admit I was relieved by my mother's change of heart because I really wanted to go where God was leading me. Even though I did not know what lay ahead of me, I had a little hope for the first time in many years that God had not abandoned me completely.

I taught at NLC from July 2002 to February 2003. The strangest thing was joining the college as a member of the faculty and being colleagues with my lecturers who had taught me while I was a B.Th. student from 1996 to 1999. I still felt like a student, and it took me some time to get used to life as a Bible college lecturer. I taught the first-year students of the bachelor's degree programme, but what was interesting was the fact that the class was a mixed group of very mature pastors, who had done certificate courses earlier and had been pastoring for many years, along with a few other young students straight out of higher secondary schools. Some students were as young as 18 and 19 years old. I also encountered a few mature students in their mid-twenties, whose parents had well-established ministries and mega-churches in the neighbouring state of Andhra Pradesh. Some of them became good friends, and I am still in touch with a few of them. I had no colleagues my age, and it was awkward trying to navigate my way around the college. What bothered me the most was some students addressing me as 'Madam', which I knew was a sign of respect, but it made me feel uncomfortable. After all, I was only 24 years old and a single woman who was still very eager to pursue higher studies.

Naga culture is similar to many Asian cultures, where great respect for the elderly and teachers is a natural component. However, while Nagas have been under the Indian constitution since Nagaland became a state of India in 1961, there are many differences in food habits and cultural traditions between the rest of India and the northeast of India. Nagas are from the Indo-Mongolian race and resemble the Burmese,

Southeast Asians, and Chinese in our facial features, food habits, dialects, and cultural aspects. For most north-eastern Indians, going to other states of India is like going to another country, requiring cultural assimilation and adjustments on many levels.

Bangalore is about 3,300 miles away from the small city I hail from in Nagaland. Even though I had spent three years in Bangalore earlier as a student, it still felt strange coming back to the city. Many things had changed in the three years I had been away. The city had expanded and developed greatly, much like some other Indian cities. Two months into my teaching, the Principal, Dr. John Thannickal, asked me to accompany a group of M.Div. students to the Asian Pentecostal Theological Conference, along with another senior colleague. It was a two-day programme and an academic affair that I was very happy to be a part of. During this conference, a group of Asian Pentecostal academicians gathered to deliberate and discuss Pentecostal Theology more academically because the usual idea that most Christians have about Pentecostalism is that Pentecostal churches have no theologians.

I was pleasantly surprised when Dr. Eim Yeol Soo from Gospel Theological Seminary (now Asia Life University) presented an interesting paper on "The Church Growth and Prayer Mountains Phenomena in South Korea." What struck me the most about his paper were the similarities between the South Korean phenomena of church growth and prayer mountains and the Indigenous Pentecostal Church in Nagaland, known as the Nagaland Christian Revival Church (NCRC), in terms of church planting and the many prayer houses set up by the NCRC believers in many corners of Nagaland from the 1970s to the present day.

During the coffee/tea break, as people were getting to know each other, I approached Dr. Eim Yeol Soo to share the similarities between South Korean Pentecostal churches and the Nagaland Christian Revival Churches. He seemed very surprised that a young woman was teaching in a Bible college and asked me my age and which country

I came from. I explained about Nagaland and how our ethnicity is different from most Indians. Since this was his first visit to India, and he had not met any Nagas before, he seemed quite surprised that Indians could look like the Chinese and Koreans. He asked if I was interested in going to GTS, Korea, to study. I told him that I was already applying to an institute in India for further studies. To my surprise, he insisted that their seminary wanted to train students from various countries in Asia and Africa.

He informed me that if I applied to study at their seminary, they would do their best to grant me a good scholarship and gave me his business card. I was quite pleasantly surprised when he told me to contact him if I ever wanted to study in South Korea. I had no intention of applying to study at their seminary, but I still thanked him. I did not think much about it until a month later when I thought it would be nice to study in a foreign country. I decided to contact Dr. Eim Yeol Soo. Just as I wrote to him for more information, I received a letter from the institute I had applied to for their Master of Theology programme in church history, saying that I was not being considered for their entrance examination. The reason was that I had only one year of experience in Christian ministry, whereas their requirement was two years of ministry experience for an applicant to the M.Th. programme.

The funny thing, though, was that I had a meeting with the then Principal of a theological institute in Bangalore, who was also its founder. What was supposed to be a 10 to 15 minutes meeting with the very respected academician cum administrator turned into an hour-long discussion on various topics, from culture to the pursuit of academic excellence and theological scholarship. I was a very ambitious woman who had completed B.Th. and M.Div. degrees and desperately wanted to pursue higher studies. Even to this day, I honestly do not know why this giant in theological education seemed impressed with me. After we discussed many topics, he assured me that I would be allowed to take the entrance examination even though the institute's requirement was two years of experience. However, I believed that God was already leading me beyond India. The Institute I am talking about is none other than the very reputed SAIACS in Bangalore and the great theological leader I was referring to is none other than the Late Dr. Graham Houghton. I carry this memory in my heart with so much gratitude because it encouraged me a great deal that someone as towering as Dr. Graham saw potential in me that I had no idea I had. I am also grateful to my colleague at NLC Dr. Bobby Varghese, an alum of SAIACS who encouraged me to meet Dr. Graham and set up an appointment for me to meet him.

Almost as soon as I wrote to Dr. Eim, I received his reply that the admissions office would contact me. True enough, I received an email from the International Admissions Office, asking me to send them my postal address so they could mail me the application forms because their website was still under construction. The application packet reached me within a week of my sending them my postal address. Since I had come to Bangalore only a month and a half after my M.Div. graduation, I had not even applied for my academic transcripts from OTS. The deadline for submission of the application was November 20, and it was already the end of October. I asked my mother in Nagaland to get my transcripts from OTS and also get the necessary recommendation letters from our local church, our tribal Baptist Association, and one from a professor at OTS. I filled in the forms and sent them to GTS from Bangalore; my mother collected the necessary documents from Nagaland and posted them to Korea.

Sometime during September 2002, I found a part-time job as a Personal Secretary to a Catholic priest at Don Bosco Centre on Hutchins Road, Bangalore. He was the Director of Don Bosco Centre. Most of the classes I taught at NLC were before noon, so I had enough time in the afternoons to keep myself busy. My work hours at the Don Bosco Centre allowed me to become friends with a few Catholic sisters. There was also a parish at the centre, and even though I did not attend any of their services or Mass, I occasionally heard young people praising and worshipping inside the parish, which surprised me because they sounded like the Protestant churches, I had grown up in. Later, I learned about the Charismatic Renewal Movement in Catholic churches that had started in Bangalore during the 1970s, especially amongst the students. I feel privileged to have known Father Sunny Uppan and Sister Josephine, whose dedication to serving God by serving His people made a profound impact on my understanding of Christian ministry. Whether a pastor or reverend in a Protestant church or a priest or nun in the Catholic Church, they are all servants of God who have responded to His call to put others first by serving them. Putting the needs of God's children above their own requires a lot of humility, surrender, and commitment. Even though I am not in contact with them anymore, I feel enriched and blessed to have known them.

I also loved working as a personal secretary because I naturally enjoyed responding to emails, posting newsletters, writing speeches, and chatting with sisters who came to Father Sunny's office whenever they needed to coordinate with him.

The winter break came and went very quickly. By February 2003, the faculty and student community of NLC were preparing for the Convocation. Two days after my 25th birthday, I received an email from Gospel Theological Seminary in Daejeon, South Korea, stating that I had been accepted into their Master of Theology programme in Church History/Historical Theology. I was assured of a full tuition scholarship and free housing. The excitement of going abroad to study was coupled with the anxiety of having to study in a country where English is not a common language. My dad seemed very nervous about the idea of sending me away. Even though he did not express his fear to me openly, I knew he did not want me to go to South Korea.

By the end of February, I went back home to Dimapur after having taught for one academic year at NLC. My health seemed better, and I was excited to volunteer for a month at the Living Bible College (LBC) in a suburb of Dimapur city. Living Bible College was started by the

Sumi NCRC, and even though I had grown up in Baptist churches, I also felt at home attending Nagaland Christian Revival Churches because my grandparents had started going to the Revival Church in the mid-1980s, and I had grown up going to their prayer centres and attending their churches every now and then with my mum.

> *"For I know the thoughts that I think toward you, says the LORD, thoughts of peace and not of evil, to give you a future and a hope."*

Jeremiah 29:11

CHAPTER 7

Healing and Understanding Missions

"Commit your way to the Lord; trust also in Him, and He shall bring it to pass."

Psalm 37:5.

Towards the end of August 2003, I left for South Korea to pursue my Master of Theology (Th.M.) in the New Testament. I was accepted to study at a small seminary known as Gospel Theological Seminary (GTS), now called Asia Life University, in the city of Daejeon. I did not know what to expect, as my only knowledge of Korea came from some Korean missionaries I had met in Bangalore while doing my bachelor's degree. However, South Korea exceeded my expectations in many ways. The kindness and generosity of Korean Christians, their spiritual discipline of fasting and intense prayers (both individual and group prayers) are examples I still talk about and admire greatly.

Their passion for world missions opened my eyes in ways I never imagined possible. The greatest challenge I faced, as do many other international students, was the need to learn Korean for better communication and survival. I also had a hard time during the first few months getting used to eating with chopsticks. Over time, I learned to relish all sorts of Korean dishes. Kimchi jjigae became my all-time favourite dish and remains so to this day. Another favourite is Bibimbap, and how can I forget the famous Korean BBQs of all kinds?

What I missed the most during my first year in Daejeon was the ability to make friends and communicate with them on a deeper level because of the language barrier. However, everyone I met at church and outside of the GTS community were very kind to me. They took the time to take me hiking, shopping, and out for lunches and dinners every now and then. The international students' community was very small, and I was the only international girl at GTS, so I felt lonely at times. However, teaching English and keeping up with assignments and paper presentations kept me busy.

To this day, I am very grateful to the professors at GTS and members of the Foursquare Church of Daejeon for the love and kindness I received from them. I want to mention Mr. Park, an English teacher at a school run by the Foursquare church of Daejeon, who went out of his way to help me find students to tutor in English so I could earn money for my necessities. While the seminary was generous enough to cover our tuition and housing, we had to pay for food, books, and other personal expenses. In many ways, I feel like my adulthood really began during my time in Korea. While I had finished two theological degrees and had already taught at my alma mater in South India before I left for Korea, I had been financially dependent on my parents until I came to Daejeon to study. The reason was that my salary in India was very little though I had not complaints about receiving a very meagre salary because the experiences and credibility I gained cannot compare to any monetary compensation. Learning to work and study at the same time was a challenge in every sense of the word; however, working part-time made me more responsible with money and helped me appreciate the life I had back home.

I was also very blessed to get to know Mr. Moon Yong Sam and his wonderful wife, Mrs. Lee. They treated me like their own daughter, going out of their way to love and bless me in every possible way. I treasure their love and friendship to this day and am so happy to still be in touch with them. Even as I write about them now, my heart is warm and filled with beautiful memories. God blessed me with wonderful friends from the International Fellowship Centre, a branch of the Foursquare Church of Daejeon. Although I cannot mention every one of them by name, a few took the time to help me get used to life in a foreign country. I am so grateful to God for providing me with friends who truly took the time to care. Anyone who has experienced living or studying in a foreign country knows how difficult it can be in the first year without a proper support system. God had everything and everyone in place for me, and I can attest to His faithfulness in truly providing for His children.

During my first semester at GTS, the student community went on a fall retreat to a mountain outside Daejeon. The fall colours took my breath away, with every tree, plant, and leaf changing to hues of orange, red, and yellow. I miss Korea even as I recollect memories of witnessing the colours and foliage for the first time. The international group and Korean language students were meeting in two different houses at the retreat centre. During a break, a Korean lady studying in the English section told me there was someone who wanted to pray for me and asked if I would be willing to receive prayers because God had revealed something to her about me. I was pleasantly surprised and willingly allowed her to pray for me. She asked if she could lay her hands on me as she prayed. The other English-speaking Korean friend translated for both of us because I couldn't understand Korean at that time and the lady praying for me couldn't understand English.

As she prayed over me, she began to tell me things that took me by surprise. She gave me words of knowledge and prophesied about things I would face in the future. The Holy Spirit revealed to her that I had a digestion problem, which was true because I had struggled with irritable bowel syndrome (IBS) and amoebic dysentery since I was a teenager. She said I would be healed from every stomach and digestion problem while in Korea. She also mentioned that I had come to Korea after facing a very difficult time, which was also true because I had experienced a heart-breaking situation a few months before coming to Daejeon. She then told me that I worried too much about my parents, which was shocking because, throughout my growing-up years, I had worried about my parents growing old. Having seen them face so many adversities and injustices, I was often very worried about them. The thought of my parents growing old was so scary to me that I often spent sleepless nights worrying. The praying lady told me to surrender my worries to God because He created my parents and would take care of them. She advised me to pray for my parents every day instead of worrying about them.

The last thing she told me was surprising, but I didn't think much about it until it came to pass six years later. She prophesied that I would marry a man who would love me very deeply. Although I had often prayed that God would provide me with a godly husband with whom I could serve Him, I did not think much about it at the time. This final prophecy came true in 2009.

God, in His faithfulness, gradually healed me from my indigestion problems, and my general health improved greatly over the next two years. I learned to pray daily for my parents and their safety. Even as my anxiety related to them decreased, I still prayed and pray for them every single day. It gave me great comfort knowing that, even as my parents have aged year after year right before my eyes, they are very much loved and cared for by their Maker, far more than I could ever care for them as their earthly daughter. God also provided me with encouraging friends who loved me with the love of Jesus Christ. I was slowly able to create many beautiful memories that helped replace the old and painful ones, although complete healing and wholeness of my soul, heart, and spirit would take many more years.

Despite all these wonderful blessings of healing and friendships, there were still days when I struggled with deep feelings of anxiety. During my third semester at GTS, I signed up for an elective class on Marriage and Family Counselling. The professor who taught the course was a brilliant counsellor and a well-known expert in Christian counselling. As the course progressed, I noticed that I had many symptoms of mental and emotional disorders that trauma patients experience. While it was a relief to realise my own need for counselling, it was very disturbing that I could not seek help because I did not know whom to approach. The professor showed slides of how our brains are affected when we face untreated trauma, and how grief can impact our bodies and minds. I began to realise that the tightening of my chest, profuse sweating of my palms, and breathlessness I often experienced before paper presentations and exams were actually panic attacks.

The whole semester was a revelation to me because, during the class, I often felt that the professor was talking about me. By the autumn of 2004, I was beginning to experience bouts of depression. Travelling to and from my part-time jobs seemed exciting at first, but after a year, juggling an intense and demanding academic programme along with part-time jobs in different places became very exhausting. I did not realise I was burning out. Towards the end of 2004, I was feeling very tired and homesick, and I just could not concentrate on my studies. While I had always been passionate about higher studies and academic rigor, I noticed a pattern of starting my academic programmes well with good grades but then ending up with lower grades towards the middle and end. History was repeating itself.

For the second time in my life, I just wanted to rest and not worry about making good grades. I wanted to be near my parents and loved ones. I was about 9,166 km away from home, and I was very tired emotionally, mentally, and physically. I took a one-week trip to Busan to visit a Naga friend who was teaching English in this beautiful city surrounded by beaches. It helped me feel a little rested. My friend, Asenla Jamir, went out of her way to make me feel welcome and loved. When I returned to Daejeon, much to the shock of my professors, friends, and parents, I made the decision to abruptly discontinue my studies. I had been applying to a few seminaries in the USA and had been accepted to a small seminary in Louisiana for a different programme, but first, I needed to go back home.

Thinking about it now breaks my heart because I felt so trapped in my own misery that I wanted to run away from all the fears, panic, pain, and dark thoughts I struggled with. Many years later, when I started therapy, I realised I had offended and deeply hurt the professors and administrative staff who had invested so much in me, a foreigner from another country, by randomly and abruptly deciding to leave the school. However, I knew deep down that I had hit rock bottom because I wasn't sleeping well at night, I couldn't concentrate on my studies, and I felt so lonely despite having a few Korean and international friends who were very kind to me. I desperately wanted to rest and have someone tell me it was okay to rest, but of course, that was not the case. I was not okay, and I would not be okay for a few more years to come.

Everyone thought I had gone mad, and a few even said it to my face. It took me a long time to realise that I wasn't in the right state of mind at that time. I had given up a good scholarship and a nurturing environment, both spiritually and academically. I felt lost, extremely tired, and very isolated. I had maintained good grades and was in my third semester, with just one more to complete my master's programme. No one in their right mind would have done what I did. However, I was so sick of the pattern of feeling very tired and wanting to give up everything every few years. I wanted to go into a deep sleep and never wake up again to deal with my exhaustion. This had happened in 1997, 1999, 2001, and then again in 2004. Despite trying very hard, I could not count my blessings. All I felt was deep sadness, dissatisfaction with myself, a lack of peace, and sheer exhaustion with life.

I vividly remember a conversation I had with my very good friend, Cha Nayoung (Esther), in the summer of 2004. I was already feeling worn out even though I did not realise it then. On a very hot summer day, we were meeting up, and I complained so much to her about my reluctance to serve God because I felt I had so many limitations. To this day, I have not forgotten what she told me, "Bokali, I have wished and prayed so many times that God would call me to serve Him full-time in Christian ministry, but He has not. That is why I teach English, but I do the best I can to serve God in whatever ways I can. You have been chosen by God to serve Him, and yet you often complain." At that point in time, I really did not feel God's presence in my life, nor did I feel called or chosen. All I felt was tiredness with my life and everything around me.

However, God was always watching over me. On my last Sunday in Daejeon, I was waiting at the office of the International Fellowship Centre (IFC) before the service started because I had come early. The IFC was a ministry started by a Nepali convert who had come to Daejeon to work but had ended up studying at GTS and co-founding the ministry of IFC with the Foursquare Church of Daejeon to reach out to migrant workers with the love of Jesus Christ. I was flipping through the pages of Isaiah when I felt my eyes rest on Isaiah 41:10: "*So do not fear, for I am with you; do not be dismayed, for I am your God. I will strengthen you and help you; I will uphold you with my righteous right hand.*" I did not hear any audible voice, but this verse really became my own. I marked it in my red leather-bound Bible and wrote down the place and the date. Somehow, I knew it was God speaking to me right there. I really did not know what lay ahead of me anymore, but I had made up my mind that I was not going to feel so tired and helpless anymore. I was going home to rest.

In November 2004, I gave up my studies (MTh.) in New Testament at Gospel Theological Seminary and headed back home to Nagaland. While I felt relieved to be home near my family, I also got into many disagreements and arguments with my mum, who could not understand why I had given up my studies in another country and come back home. At that time, I felt hurt that my mum did not understand my need to make my own decisions. Today, I fully understand her frustration with me for giving up my studies. The frustration of not being able to explain my struggles with depression was very painful. I felt useless and angry at myself again for not being able to live up to my family's expectations, especially my mum's. I felt like a complete failure. I did not know what to do next. While a very big part of me wanted to just stay home and be with my parents, it was unthinkable for me to let my parents go through the disappointment of having a daughter who was a failure and a drop-out from a seminary in another country.

So, it was a miracle when a kind Korean friend, Mr. GW Choi from IFC, offered to help me out by inviting me to Korea on a visitor's visa.

By February 2005, I left for South Korea again. God opened the way for me to get admission to Seoul Christian University in the spring of 2005. A month after regular classes had started, I was allowed to transfer only 12 credits from my previous seminary, so I had to practically repeat my second year and complete the Korean language course too. However, I was very grateful and relieved to be able to continue with my studies again.

Embarking on a journey as a student in the city of Seoul was very interesting. God took care of me as He had always done.

> *"The LORD is good, A stronghold in the day of trouble; And He knows those who trust in Him."*
>
> Nahum 1:7.

CHAPTER 8

Miracle in Seoul – My Nineveh Experience

"I can do all things through Christ who strengthens me."

Philippians 4:13.

Life in Seoul was quite different from life in Daejeon. There were many more international students and professionals from various countries in Seoul than in Daejeon. This meant I could communicate with many more people in English and make friends more easily. Since I did not get a room at the dorm during my first semester, owing to my very late acceptance at Seoul Christian University, I lived with a Naga friend who kindly allowed me to share her place. I had to get used to living in a new place all over again, but this time, despite the regular difficulties of moving, I felt much more at peace because there were quite a few Naga brothers and sisters in the greater Seoul area. Living in Seoul helped me mature and realise that if we set our minds to do anything and do it sincerely, we can survive anywhere in the world. Living in Seoul also made me experience God's provision in unexpected and life-changing ways. I met and made friends who were very kind to me when I least expected their kindness.

One of the main things my family prayed for before I left for South Korea to study in 2003 was that God would provide me with good friends. Even though I believed God would provide me with good friends, He exceeded all my expectations because He provided me with amazing friends in Daejeon and Seoul, who loved me, cared for me, and took care of me as my own family would. During my first semester at Seoul Christian University, I was introduced to a youthful woman named Kim JH by a mutual friend. JH and I bonded over an American accent neutralisation course we both attended. Even though we are no longer in touch, I am so grateful to God for sending her to be a great blessing to me. She took me shopping, taught me to be smart with money, introduced me to a church that hired me as their pastor for a small English congregation on Sunday afternoons, and introduced me to another amazing friend, Mr. Michael Putlack. Mr. Michael is an American English Lecturer, and a writer who was a great blessing to me throughout my year of studies in Seoul and later when I moved to America. Michael is now married and has relocated to Thailand, but to this day, he has been a blessing to a small, faith-based non-profit organisation that I run with my mum to reach out to women living below the poverty line in Dimapur, the city I now live in.

Another family and ministry that God used to train me in Seoul was Rev. Moon and his family at Withee Mission International (WMI), based in Ansan City, south of Seoul. Rev. Moon's passion and ministry towards the migrant workers' community in the greater Seoul area opened my eyes to the opportunities of doing missions wherever we are, especially in our own backyards and alleys instead of always thinking of missions as going overseas (though I know the importance of overseas mission work is greater than ever now, with the world having become a global village). Seeing Korean churches reach out to foreigners in their own land enabled me to understand the need to reach out to my own brothers and sisters back home and to the many non-Naga communities that have migrated and settled in Nagaland. During the autumn of 2004, I began to develop a desire to do missions through social work. I had grown up in a very conservative Christian family, and even after years of studying in Bible colleges and seminaries, my understanding of Christian missions and ministry was strictly confined to classroom instructions in a theological college or seminary, being a clergy, or working for a Christian organisation.

My association with Rev. Moon and WMI started in 2004. When I was still a student in Daejeon, I met Rev. Moon at a Missions Workshop in the spring of 2004 and was surprised to meet a Korean Reverend who seemed to know about Nagaland and the Nagas very well. It turned out he had been to Nagaland a few times and desired to train and work with Naga Christians.

From the spring of 2005 till the summer of 2006, I taught at the weekend Bible college at WMI and had the opportunity to fellowship at San Somang Church, also known as Living Hope International Church, pastored by Rev. Moon every Sunday morning. As my Master's in Theology programme was coming to an end, I had no plans to immediately return home to Nagaland.

I desired to stay and work in Daejeon or Seoul for a year while applying for doctoral studies at seminaries or universities in Korea or elsewhere. I did not spend enough time praying about my next steps after graduation. However, in my mind, I had already decided I wanted to stay in Korea and work for a year. I desperately wanted a break from my studies since I had been studying for many years. However, God had another adventure planned for me.

In March 2006, shortly after returning to Korea from the winter break at home in Nagaland, I began to experience severe anxiety. I was often very tired, had trouble sleeping at night, and did not want to wake up in the mornings. I had gone through this experience in the past and, as usual, I blamed myself for my anxieties. I felt a lump on the right side of my neck and began to have severe headaches as well as pain in the same side of my ears and neck. I was writing my final thesis and struggled to concentrate. Between April and June, I made ten visits to two different hospitals. I was diagnosed with a thyroid tumour and, even though it was benign, I was still alarmed. The medications left me utterly drained. Taking five different tablets, three times a day, meant I was consuming fifteen tablets daily, leaving me exhausted beyond words. I lost a lot of weight, and the swelling on my neck made me feel very uncomfortable, frustrated, and sad. I felt disoriented during the day and very tired both emotionally and physically. At times, I felt like I was floating in my body.

The trips to the hospital were quite lonely because I went alone most of the time, except for one occasion when a Pakistani friend named Nadeem Raja accompanied me. I remain grateful to him to this day for helping a sister in need. Raja was also a student at Presbyterian College and Theological Seminary (PCTS) in Seoul. I had come to know Raja through a dear Naga sister, Kaisa Kayina, who remains a close friend. The three of us spent many weekends together, eating and watching Bollywood movies. Raja had a massive collection of Indian movies, and, though I grew up in India, I had never been a Bollywood fan. Thanks to Raja, I began to watch Hindi movies and started introducing them to my Korean friends as well.

Recollecting these small but memorable experiences reminds me of the lifelong and meaningful friendships formed far away from home. Our shared experiences as foreigners, our struggles with a new culture, different perspectives, learning new things, unlearning a few, and bonding over food helped us overcome homesickness and loneliness. Friends become family in this kind of environment, and I was blessed to find a strong support system in friends who were there for me. The Naga community in Seoul was a great blessing to me. I started watching Korean dramas for the first time when I met sister Zakani (whom I fondly call Afo Zaka), with whom I still maintain a very close relationship. We started watching a Korean drama series, "My Lovely Kim Sam Soon" (MNKSM), which was very popular in Korea at that time. Afo Zaka and I became fans of the series. Since there were about seven of us Nagas studying at SCU, along with a few other Indian friends from other states, we relied on each other. I remember other Naga sisters and brothers with the fondest memories, thinking back to our outings and annual meetings at Dr. Kenny Kapfo's and his wife Dr. Paulah's house every few months. Hanging out with them always made me feel like I was home in Nagaland.

Since I was already in my final semester, an elderly friend in Daejeon introduced me to a pastor of a medium-sized church with about 1,500 congregation members. They were willing to help sponsor me for a missionary visa to stay in Korea after my graduation. I visited Daejeon towards the end of spring, despite my poor health. There, I met with the senior pastor to finalise our plan for me to work there after my graduation, starting in the summer of 2006. However, even after nearly two months of medication, I felt increasingly stressed and worn out. During one of my final trips to the hospital towards the end of my semester, I was advised to undergo surgery to remove my thyroid. Being far from home and having already had two surgeries on my throat (one at seven years old and another at nineteen), I did not want to proceed without my family around me.

I had to make a very difficult decision immediately. Since I was only a couple of months away from completing my course, I decided to go home. My plan was to rest and be with my parents for a year before planning for further studies. Although my heart was not ready to leave Seoul, a city I had grown to love for its vibrant, hi-tech, and fast-paced nature, I felt it was best for me to go home and rest.

During my first year in South Korea, I faced the usual cultural and language difficulties that foreigners encounter in a new country. By the second year, I had made a few good friends and had become more comfortable, adjusting to many new things, including my love for Korean food and occasional window shopping to de-stress. By the third year, I was becoming proficient in basic conversational Korean, passing my Hangeul exam, and enjoying socialising with friends. However, it was time for me to leave. While I trusted that God knew what was best for me, my heart felt heavy and sad about leaving Seoul. I still think of South Korea with the fondest memories and hope to visit again soon.

I cannot forget is the natural beauty of Korean spring and autumn colours. Every plant and tree blooms in spring, and they change colours in the autumn season. I also discovered that, while it was not easy juggling full-time studies and part-time work, it was possible, and I enjoyed being financially independent. Though I could not afford a luxurious lifestyle, I was able to pay my own bills and go shopping occasionally. This was quite liberating and empowering for someone who had lived a very dependent life until a few years ago.

Even though my plans did not work out, God, in His amazing ways, allowed me to experience complete healing of my thyroid tumour within a week of my decision to go home. Rev. Moon had been encouraging me for about six months to return to Nagaland to work as their Coordinator for the new Withee Missions Office they were planning to start. When I decided to go home and my thyroid tumour disappeared within a week, I knew that God was watching over me. Rev. Moon told me that I had been running like the prophet Jonah, who did not want to preach at Nineveh. I understood what he meant. I knew then that God had an assignment for me back home. I was curious about how He would lead me, but I trusted that He would never disappoint me.

> *"And my God shall supply all your need according to His riches in glory by Christ Jesus."*
>
> Philippians 4:19.

CHAPTER 9

Mission Naga

"Peace I leave with you, My peace I give to you; not as the world gives do I give to you. Let not your heart be troubled, neither let it be afraid."

John 14:27.

I had to leave Korea and return to Nagaland to allow my body to rest. On the bright side, a new chapter awaited me back home. When I returned in August, I began working as a Missions Coordinator for Withee Mission International's branch office in my home city, Dimapur. My job was to coordinate with the head office in Ansan City, South Korea, to start a professional Missions Conference called Mission Naga – patterned after the Mission Korea Conferences held in South Korea every other year. Mission Korea is a professional Missions Conference attended by thousands of Korean missionaries serving all over the world, co-organised by multiple mission organisations.

From October, I had to start operating from our small office in Dimapur. I first appointed two staff members, mobilised volunteers, organised Concerts of Prayer in different Bible colleges and churches with youths, and hosted Korean Pre-Mission teams every few months, leading up to the Mission Naga Conference in July 2007. Starting anything new is quite challenging, and even though I knew the task ahead would not be easy, I was aware that this was where God wanted me to be at that point in time. He proved faithful every step of the way.

Putting together a committee to organise Mission Naga 2007, setting up a prayer committee, finding a venue, and trying to introduce the concept of starting a professional mission conference in a Christian state where every church and tribal association has its own mission projects and conferences, proved to be more daunting than I had ever imagined. Many well-intentioned friends and very respected senior leaders in ministry tried to discourage me from organising an independent conference. However, after attending two Mission Korea Conferences in 2004 and 2006, my eyes and heart were open to the idea and need to educate young people about approaching and carrying out missions from various perspectives.

Most Naga Christians still view being a missionary as the job of a theological or Bible school graduate, but the Great Commission of Jesus is for His disciples to preach the gospel in our own back and front yards, in the marketplaces, and to nations far and wide. This kind of mission calls for all disciples of Christ, from every profession, to be missionaries in whatever capacity they can serve and minister the message of the gospel of Jesus Christ.

Until I left for South Korea to study, my understanding of being a missionary was limited to facing persecutions, financial worries, and going to states or countries with unreached people groups (countries with populations among which there are few or no indigenous Christians). I had met a few medical missionary doctors and nurses, and quite a few Christians from professional music backgrounds becoming missionaries. However, studying in South Korea and witnessing Korean churches doing missions with great zeal, passion, and creativity broadened my perspective on missions, both locally and overseas.

Being associated with Withee Mission International and its founder, Rev. Barnabas C. Moon, helped me understand the importance of reaching out to migrant workers in my own country. I was blessed to teach at the weekend Bible school for migrant workers at Withee Headquarters in Ansan City, south of Seoul. The students at the weekend Bible school were migrant workers from many African countries and Southeast Asia, who came to work in the factories and industrial estates of South Korea.

Withee HQ also hosted African community worship services, and I was privileged to become friends with quite a few African brothers and sisters from Nigeria, Cameroon, and Ghana. Worshipping with the African community was like attending a concert with foot-tapping and, often, dancing. Many of these migrant workers came to work in South Korea to make a living but would return to their own countries and become missionaries in partnership with Korean churches and ministries after acquiring a newfound commitment to the message of Jesus Christ and gaining more knowledge about world missions.

These new insights on migrant worker missions, an ever-increasing personal curiosity about what God wanted the churches in Nagaland to be a part of, and a desire to create awareness for graduates about the available opportunities led me to be part of the Mission Naga Conference, which began humbly in 2007 at Eastern Bible College during a very hot summer week. Many gifted men and women of God sacrificed their time and resources to help make the first-ever Mission Naga 2007 conference a success. The Western Sumi Baptist Akukuhou Kuqhakulu (WSBAK) partnered with Withee Mission International, and the NMM (Nagaland Missions Movement) helped organise different sub-events during the five-day conference. Rev. Vitoshe Swu, the Executive Director of WSBAK at that time, and Rev. Dr. Anjo Keikong, the then Director of NMM, both went out of their way to support and help ensure the successful conduct of the first-ever Mission Naga.

Dr. Tereso Casino, from Torch Trinity Graduate School of Theology (now Torch Trinity Graduate University) in Seoul, South Korea, was the main speaker at the conference. Several local and national mission organisations set up booths to inform participants about mission opportunities and the work being done by them in India and beyond. Around 33 volunteers from South Korea and the UK came to assist in organising and managing Mission Naga 2007, serving as resource persons for seminars, counselling sessions, and more.

Eastern Bible College graciously offered their facilities for the conference, and their students and faculty helped as volunteers. Mr. David Khobung and his wife, Alibo, kindly let us use their staff quarters for many months leading up to the conference. It was there that we had numerous meals and cups of tea over meetings and prayers. The Founder and Principal of EBC, the Late Dr. T.M. Lotha, who has now gone to be with the Lord, will be remembered for EBC's historical significance as the first venue used to train young Naga people for missions.

By June 2007, I had been accepted into Boston University's School of Theology for a Master of Sacred Theology programme. I applied for another master's programme because applying for doctoral programmes intimidated me. After wrapping up Mission Naga 2007 at the end of July, I started my visa application for Boston. Although I had heard many stories about the difficulty of obtaining an American visa, I was pleasantly surprised to find that my visa interview lasted only a few minutes, and I was granted a five-year visa for a two-year programme.

Everything happened very quickly, and by the end of August 2007, I left for America with a lot of positive expectations, not knowing that great challenges and more painful times lay ahead. Had I known of the darker times and the pain I would face, I might not have left the security of my family and home.

"The Lord is my shepherd; I shall not want."

Psalm 23:1.

CHAPTER 10

Boston, USA

"…casting all your care upon Him, He cares for you."
1 Peter 5:7.

I arrived in the United States of America during the autumn season as a new international student at the Boston University School of Theology (BUSTH). The journey from Nagaland to Boston was long, and it took me a while to adjust to the time difference between India and America. I had travelled from Mumbai to JFK, New York, and by the time I landed at JFK airport for a short layover before boarding a plane to Boston, I felt like a zombie. I still remember my ride from Boston's Logan International Airport to my dorm at Newton Centre on the Andover Newton Theological School campus (ANTS).

The cab driver and I engaged in casual conversation. When I told him it was my first time in America, he seemed shocked because I spoke fluent English. He told me his name was Nehemiah, and he was from Haiti. When I arrived at the ANTS campus, a student who was already living in the building where I was assigned helped me with my luggage. His name was Alex, and he also seemed very surprised that I spoke fluent English. I had to keep explaining to everyone I met that I hail from a hilly state in the northeast of India, that our people are from the Indo-Mongolian race, that I hold a valid Indian passport, and that English is the official language of Nagaland even though we have our tribal dialects. I had to repeat this conversation to nearly everyone I met for the first time over the next three years of my stay in Boston.

Another amusing experience was being mistaken for a Korean or Chinese during my first week at BUSTH. I made an effort to acknowledge Korean students by greeting them with a bow, as they do in Korea. Sometimes, I even said, *"Anyeong haseyo"* (a Korean greeting) to them. Except for a few with whom I had already spoken, many mistook me for a Korean for a couple of months. I smile at the memory even as I write about it. I felt much loved and welcomed by my new Korean friends, who sometimes invited me to their gatherings, where I enjoyed Korean food to my heart's content. I also attended English Bible study at a Korean church every Thursday evening, not far from the campus where I lived. I met some wonderful friends who went out of their way to welcome me. I remain very grateful to my friend and brother, Dr. Sangduk Kim, for introducing me to his church and for being a faithful brother in Christ throughout our years of study together at BUSTH.

Despite being able to connect with Korean friends and hang out with them, I realised that getting used to life in a new country and culture is never easy. I didn't know how hard and lonely life could be as an international student in America. During my first semester at BU, just a month after arriving in Boston, I began to experience extreme anxiety, sleeplessness, loss of appetite, and other symptoms of depression. I had often struggled with these symptoms in the past, but as I mentioned earlier, I often blamed myself for being fearful and weak. In the past, I had managed to survive by trying to appear normal in front of others and getting on with my life. Looking back now, I realise I was able to cope with emotional breakdowns in the past because I was in Asia. I will explain why my coping mechanisms crashed completely in this completely alien environment.

Most Asian societies are very community oriented. While this can sometimes feel suffocating, we are generally less individualistic than in Western cultures. I mention this not to compare but to explain a realisation I had many years later: while struggling with depression, I somehow felt watched over by friends or family. In America, however, I was practically alone most of the time, even though a Naga family and a few good friends reached out to me during my first month and semester. People in America were less intrusive about personal lives, with everyone going about their own business without much concern for others. In a way, it was liberating; I once told an American friend on campus that I felt like I could breathe in peace without constantly worrying about being answerable to those who judged me or gave unsolicited advice.

Despite my feelings of alienation and isolation, God was still watching over me, sending guardian angels to help. Dr. Mar Imsong and his wife, Bendangla Jamir, with their three children, became like family to me from my first month in Boston. They had heard about a Naga girl coming to Boston University to study and came to find me one evening at my dorm at ANTS in Newton Centre, a suburb about a 30-minute train ride from Boston University. Although I was a BUSTH student, both ANTS and BUSTH were members of the Boston Theological Institute (BTI), a consortium of theological and divinity schools in the greater Boston area, including the Harvard Divinity School. BTI students could live on each other's campuses, access each other's libraries, and enrol in classes at any BTI member school.

Dr. Mar Imsong was then the senior pastor of the First Baptist Church of Bedford, Concord MA, about a 40 to 45-minute drive from my dorm. I started attending their church regularly and became a member for a year and a half. I am forever grateful to Dr. Imsong, his family, and the congregation of FBC Bedford for their love, hospitality, and acceptance. I will never forget leading worship every Sunday, singing with Joan the pianist, practising with Laureen, and fellowshipping with Linda and Mike over lunch after church. My love for Boston's clam chowder began the first Sunday at FBC when

Mike and Linda took me to lunch after the service – a tradition that soon developed. I was also greatly surprised and touched when FBC Bedford gifted me a new laptop in my first month there, even before I became a member. Over the next two years, Dr. Mar Imsong and FBC Bedford played crucial roles in helping me receive book grants and a continuing education scholarship from TABCOM (The American Baptist Churches of Massachusetts). I am also very grateful to Twila Wannamaker of FBC Bedford for the wonderful recommendation letter she wrote, which allowed me to receive another scholarship from the Women's Department of TABCOM.

While I had this wonderful and supportive church family to rely on during weekends, weekdays were very hard. I had to commute to school by train, work part-time at BU West Campus' Dining Services, and juggle assignments and readings. I had little time to meet and make new friends, except for classmates who seemed equally busy, if not more so. Every other student I knew was struggling like me, juggling studies with part-time jobs. Boston is a very expensive city and worrying about surviving my first year only added to my anxiety.

I arrived in Boston in late August 2007, and by October, I was in deep depression. I never really thought anyone would understand my struggles, so I didn't tell anybody about my panic attacks, the pains and aches in my body, heavy-headedness, or the difficulty waking up in the mornings. As I had done in the past, I kept my depressive thoughts, sleepless nights, and constant fear to myself, doing my best to cope with and suppress my deep pain and extreme depression.

I thought I was doing a good job of surviving breakdowns by forcing myself to function, but this time, a few new friends began to notice my depression.

I noticed in America there was a higher awareness of mental health issues compared to my home region. People I met seemed more psychologically aware and talked openly about mental health struggles, medication, and therapy. In my psychology and counselling courses in India and South Korea, it was uncommon for people to openly discuss these issues. Thankfully, today, with social media and celebrities discussing mental health, there is increased awareness and more trained professionals, even in Nagaland.

One evening, on a train ride back to campus, I met another BU international student from Zimbabwe, who later became a good friend. She told me, "Boka, you do not look normal to me. You seem to be struggling with depression, which is common for most international students who come to America to study." She advised me to share my struggles with the Dean of Students at the School of Theology and seek professional help. Throughout my first semester, I was blessed with a few friends who reached out to me, bringing much healing to my heart, and helping me deal with trust issues from past relationships.

Nicole Long and Emilia Halstead, my dorm neighbours at the Appleton Chase Building, reached out to me with kindness and love, helping me realise I was not alone. I will forever be grateful to Nicole for helping me find a part-time job, which I needed for financial survival in the first semester. She also gifted me a beautiful potted plant in the first month. Emilia was a true sister, who loved me, protected me, made me laugh, cheered me up, and loaned me DVDs for relaxation.

Ramona Guadalupe, a godly woman from Vermont studying at ANTS, invited me to her student apartment every Thursday for dinner and prayer. These wonderful ladies helped me experience divine love in ways that brought healing to my wounded spirit. My heart was shredded beyond repair over several years.

Taking my friend's advice from the train ride and another friend's suggestion about a mental health clinic at the university, I went to the Danielsen Institute, a multidisciplinary mental health clinic at Boston University. I don't quite remember if it was the end of

October or early November, but winter had not yet set in, though it was already very chilly. I will always remember my walk from BU's East Campus to Bay State Road, feeling lost and isolated, my heart broken, wondering what had become of me. Here I was, a 29-year-old educated woman, pursuing her third master's degree at a world-class university, having travelled halfway around the world to America, yet feeling utterly messed up. I wondered if I would ever find healing and wholeness. Despite the chill I felt in my body as well as in my spirit, I still remember looking at the beautiful orange and yellow leaves that was falling off the trees lining up Baystate Road.

Back home, my family thought highly of me, and my church and community believed I had it all together. Yet, here I was, so confused that I did not even know who I was anymore. What made it worse was that I had chosen to pursue theological studies with the hope of working in Christian ministry, serving God and people. I felt broken and ashamed of my brokenness. The hardest part was admitting that I felt so useless. Even though I had experienced major emotional breakdowns before, this time I was almost unable to function. I did not want to be around anyone, so I would just attend my classes in a blur, head to work, and then return to my dorm. I wanted to eat alone, be left alone, and exist as if I were invisible. There were days when I could not even get out of bed and had to miss classes.

What scared me the most was the thought that I could never truly minister or reach out to others because I was so broken and could not function normally. I struggled with the thought that I had nothing to offer anyone, leading to suicidal thoughts. Although I had experienced the desire to die before, this time the thought of taking my own life occurred daily. I have no adequate words to describe the hellish experience of living in such darkness, which lasted through the autumn of 2007, while I was doing my first semester at Boston University School of Theology.

I confided in my mum over the phone about my depression, and she began to tell me that, as born-again, spirit-filled Christians, depression should have no place in our lives. While I had always admired my mother's ability to give all her problems to the Lord and retain her sanity despite experiencing so much trauma and negativity, I could not be like her. It seemed to hurt her that I was not as strong as she was. Although I love my mother very much, it hurt me that the one person I needed to support me always seemed to judge me. However, now I know that Mum never stopped interceding for me, and for that, I am very grateful. I am thankful to God for a mother who never lets a day go by without praying for her children and family.

During the long walk to the Danielsen Institute, I experienced loneliness, shame, and every other negative feeling. After filling out forms, being matched with a competent and gifted therapist, and sorting out the payment method with my medical insurance, I was ready to start a journey toward healing, even though I didn't know what to expect at the time. I still remember the first time I stepped into my therapist's office. His name was Dr. David Goodman. I was so nervous and still very depressed, feeling as if someone outside of me was doing the talking. My real self-seemed dead inside; I was just a shell of my former self. I remember being asked a few questions about myself and how I was feeling, but I don't recall all the details from my first counselling session with Dr. Goodman. I was desperate to find healing and did my best during our interactions over the following months.

After a few sessions, Dr. Goodman diagnosed me with clinical depression. Medically, this meant I had a severe form of depression known as Major Depressive Disorder. My symptoms included persistent depression, deep sadness, fixation on past mistakes and failures, self-recrimination for perceived mistakes, loss of appetite, feelings of worthlessness, suicidal thoughts, extreme anxiety, and panic attacks – all of which had been part of my life for the past decade.

It took me months to realise how ill I had been for so many years. I often wonder what would have become of me had I not gone to

Boston University when I did. To this day, I recognise the hand of God and His perfect timing in allowing me to receive the help I desperately needed. I am grateful that I had the time and resources available in America to find restoration and healing in ways I could never have imagined. It would not be an exaggeration to say that it was Dr. Goodman, during my two years of therapy, who helped me rediscover parts of myself I thought I had lost forever. He helped me understand the meaning of depression and the reasons behind it. Most importantly, my therapy sessions made me see that there truly was light at the end of a very long and dark tunnel.

Even so, I needed to take things one day at a time. There were many days when I felt that going to therapy was pointless because my life did not seem worth living. Breakthroughs did not happen overnight, but having someone listen to me, help me express my fears, talk about years of bottled-up feelings, and not make me feel weak or tell me to be strong helped me regain my self-respect and self-worth. The process was slow but empowering. I was assured that it was okay to feel weak and helpless and that I was not alone in my mental health struggles. With help, I could actually manage my emotions better. If I was willing to go through the difficult process of finding and resolving issues I needed to work on, there could be healing and wholeness – even if it took time, maybe even a lifetime.

I was grateful to be reminded repeatedly that therapy was about seeking healing and wholeness. This was possible if I was willing to face my fears, be honest about my control issues and anger towards myself and others, and let go of many toxic emotions. Therapy opened my eyes to the fact that mental illness is like any other illness, even though we don't see visible scars or injuries. I understood that we should never hesitate to seek help from mental health experts, professionals, spiritual mentors, or prayer partners who will not judge us. Listening to music with uplifting lyrics and words of hope helped me feel a little less depressed because it made me feel understood in my brokenness, darkness, and helplessness.

Over the following year, Dr. Goodman helped me arrange a meeting with a psychiatrist on campus, who prescribed medication for six months to manage my depression and insomnia. I did not want to be dependent on pills, so I did my best to take care of myself and stay occupied. I wrote down small goals to achieve each day, even though consistency was difficult. The most important lesson I learned during my therapy was to take time to care for myself, live in the moment, and take one day at a time.

I felt the hand of the divine in many small things and experiences that brought me joy in unexpected ways. Taking long walks, praying, and having long phone conversations with girlfriends and Naga sisters living in different parts of America brought me calm. To this day, I have a close bond with my sister and dear friend, Afo Akhuli Zhimo, who lives in Florida. We share a strong connection because of our shared experiences with physical and emotional challenges. Another friend, Khati Prosonic from Syracuse, always loved and accepted me, blessed me, and reached out to me in a way that makes me feel like the most blessed person on earth.

It was a huge relief to find out that many people faced and lived with emotional and mental issues like me. We have to learn to seek help. It is imperative that we obtain help from professionals if we ever wanted to get back on our feet and live a functional life.

Even after starting the process, I found it physically and mentally exhausting to work part-time, study, and start a new life in Boston. Initially, Boston seemed like an old colonial city that was slow-paced. I couldn't help but compare it to the high-tech, fast-paced city of Seoul. Slowly, I discovered that Boston was a busy city too. It grew on me, and over the years I lived there, I came to love it.

I began my therapy with one session every Thursday. Later, my therapist felt it would be better to have two sessions a week. On days when I was having panic attacks or extreme anxiety, I could call my therapist for an emergency session. Sometimes, I met with my therapist three times a week. There were days when I honestly thought I would never see a time when I could manage or live with the unseen demons in my head. Dying seemed like the only option to escape the pain and torture. I was very angry with myself many days because I wanted to be in control, but clearly, I was not.

On one particularly hard day, as I was still struggling to function normally and identify my issues, Dr. Goodman asked me to go home and write a letter to my 19-year-old self and bring it to him the following week. So, I returned to my dorm and wrote a few pages to myself. I was surprised at how therapeutic it was to address myself as if I were someone else. I told 'myself' to forgive others and forgive myself, and that her life mattered to many people. I was also surprised to see that I could write about the fact that life is never easy for anyone and that unexpected tragedies happen to many families, not just mine. I had lived for years thinking my family alone had suffered pain, injustice, shame, and sad experiences that didn't always have answers. I was also able to express hope for the future, which was truly comforting. After writing the long letter, I re-read it many times before taking it to my therapist. He made me read it out to him. It felt surreal yet liberating to detach myself from all the tangled, destructive emotions I had felt for so many years and realise I didn't have to define myself by those toxic, negative emotions. I felt like I was finally stepping away from a war zone to a more peaceful place. Writing the letter was a life-changing experience and a significant breakthrough in my healing journey. I kept the letter for some time but eventually burnt it after a few months, as was my tradition with journals.

Even though I spiralled back into depression many times after experiencing days of feeling lighter and better, I began to truly understand mental illness. Regular therapy sessions, learning healing practices, and sticking to them helped me confront many big and small issues that had lived in my thoughts and mind for so long. Some of these practices included taking deep breaths and calming myself by talking to myself during panic attacks, listening to uplifting music and motivational speakers (mostly Christian speakers who had gone through brokenness themselves), and calling someone I knew I could talk to when plagued with negative and repetitive thoughts. I realised that there were spiritual strongholds in my life that could only be broken by developing new thinking patterns. This change could be brought about by constantly reading and meditating on God's word to help renew my mind.

I also began to slowly open up to a few friends who were able to talk to me over the phone when I started to feel depressed and helpless. Heidi Montero, a very good, committed Christian girl, became my friend during one of my trips to Yonkers, New York. She was always there for me, praying with me, and encouraging me over the phone. My cousin's wife, Lovily, who lived in Fort Worth, Texas, listened to me every week over the phone and prayed with me. These ladies were angels who showed me so much love and reached out to me with such grace that my life has been forever changed. Lovily remains a good friend and sister who prays for me even at midnight when I need immediate help and prayers. My healing journey was greatly impacted by these beautiful women of God.

I coined my own term for my deep depression – I called it an 'emotional dungeon'. It was a very dark place that seemed like a bottomless pit, going deeper and deeper with each breakdown every year. For many years, there seemed to be no hope for me, no light at the end of that deep and dark tunnel. However, that began to change as I learned and realised that I had been mentally ill. With the right diagnosis, therapy, medication, and a lot of love and support from friends, I found healing and recovery.

I was also very blessed to be part of the Graduate Christian Fellowship (GCF) at Boston University. GCF is part of InterVarsity Fellowship, a campus ministry that reaches out to students worldwide. Tim Leary and his wife, Sarah Leary, have been ministering to American and international students like me at Boston University. I have beautiful memories of fellowshipping with the Bible study group of GCF in the basement of Marsh Chapel every Wednesday and going to dinner with the group. Fellowshipping with this group built me up spiritually in ways I never knew I needed. I also learned to intentionally take time out for myself, treat myself to leisure walks and meet friends or hang out over coffee or tea in Boston's many beautiful areas. These small weekly traditions did my heart good because I felt valued while being around friends who genuinely cared about me.

While studying at Bible colleges and seminaries, I had unknowingly developed the thought that I knew everything about faith, the Word, and anything spiritual. Looking back now, I feel sad that I had not dealt with my pride. Studying the scriptures with students from different fields of study at BU, who were born again, hungry for the Word of God, believed in evangelism, and cared about me and my well-being, made me truly understand the importance and value of being part of a Christian community that embodies the love of Jesus in a very real way. While I am very grateful for my theological education and the degrees I have earned, I can say without hesitation that the greatest blessings from my years in Boston are the friendships that allowed me to grow, heal, and understand that Jesus died for me to recreate me in His image and likeness. Because of this, my sole aspiration today is to try to be more like Jesus – to be more kind, gentle, loving, and understanding, as He was to everyone who sought Him.

I've often struggled to be a perfectionist in my own abilities, trying to live a sanctified life in my thoughts and actions, but met with constant failures. The spiritual concept of Victorious Christian Living was a very hard standard to live up to. Only by completely surrendering to Jesus, acknowledging my human inability and limitations, was I able to rely on the strength provided by the Holy Spirit as promised by Jesus in the Gospels and through lived experiences as written in the epistles of St. Paul in the New Testament.

Even as I write this, I cannot help but feel truly grateful and amazed that today, I can talk and write about my years of depression, panic attacks, and suicidal thoughts as if they happened to someone else. I have come a long way from the scarred, bruised, angry, and battered girl I was many years ago. I know that not everyone who seeks professional help finds healing and wholeness as I did. Some live the rest of their lives without fully recovering, some learn to manage, while others succumb to their struggles, and some even take their own lives. I can only say that depression does not control me anymore. I have truly found healing and deliverance from the demons that tortured me for years.

While I did not have hallucinations, I did have terrible recurring dreams for many years. I did not hear anything clearly, but there were many noises and crazy thoughts in my head about myself and what others thought of me. I lived in constant fear of what others were saying about me, obsessing over my failures and mistakes, and fixating on what had happened to my family and my life. I spent so much energy on negative thoughts and fear that it was impossible for me to enjoy the blessings I had right before me. I could not take healthy pride in any of my achievements.

Even though I knew deep down that I needed help when I first sought out the Danielsen Institute, I did not realise the extent of my problems' toxicity. There were layers of emotions I had not dealt with. Digging them out one by one was not only very uncomfortable and extremely painful, but it felt like toxic bombs of emotions were bursting out of my heart, soul, and spirit. I was often exhausted, both physically and emotionally. There were days when I felt on top of the world after a breakthrough session with my therapist (which was not very often), but the next day, I would be down in the dumps, feeling lonely, with darkness clouding my thoughts and emotions. I barely sat through every class I signed up for during my first and second semesters at BUSTH. Thankfully, I did not fail any classes, but I did not achieve any As in my first year.

There came a time when I had to take my Zimbabwean friend's advice and meet the Dean of Students about my mental health. This was sometime before the winter break. The patient and empathetic attention I received from the Dean, Dr. Shiela Imani, surprised me. She told me that if I did not love myself, I would never be able to give love or minister to anyone after my studies. She advised me to focus on my healing and wholeness. It felt like a light had dawned on me after a very long, extremely dark journey. To this day, I feel so grateful and blessed that God brought me to America at that time. The restoration I received in every area of my life and the help and support I needed to find healing and wholeness would not have happened had I not gone to Boston University.

In the midst of all this, I was very blessed to have my cousin and his wife living in Fort Worth, Texas. They graciously invited me to spend my first Thanksgiving holidays in America with them. My cousin, Khetoshe Chishi (Akheto), and I had attended Patkai Christian College in Nagaland together for two years, bonding like real siblings during those years. We had kept in touch over the years, even though we had gone to different places to continue our studies. In 2003, when I went to South Korea to study, Akheto married a beautiful Sumi lady named Lovily Vito Sema in Dallas, Texas. Although they were neighbours in Nagaland, they met and fell in love in Texas.

Lovily and I were first introduced to each other over email by Akheto. Though we met for the first time in 2007, I felt very welcomed, loved, and accepted by Lovily. They had a beautiful three-year-old daughter named Elsheli, who seemed rather grown-up for her age. Even though I had known Lovily over emails and phone calls for about five years, meeting her in person was amazing. We had so much to talk about. For the first time in many years, I felt like I wasn't alone. She seemed to read my mind, understand my depressive thoughts and my instability, which I had tried so hard to hide for so many years. I had not realised it until then. During a conversation alone in their guest room, I started to cry over something she had noticed about me. She saw that I was broken, struggling with self-esteem issues and trust issues, and trying very hard to keep it all together.

I was shocked that I was crying in front of someone, especially a female friend because I had never done that before. Meeting her, interacting with her, and having her minister to me with unconditional love and acceptance made me feel liberated and accepted in a way I had never felt before. I allowed myself to be loved and accepted. Even though I grew up with many wonderful girlfriends and had many from the colleges and seminaries I attended, facing this darkness of a mental and emotional breakdown, and unearthing my hurts and scars bit by bit took me by surprise because my emotions were so unstable.

One of the things I discovered about myself during that Thanksgiving break was that I had never really let go of the hurt an older female friend caused me back in 1997, while I was a student in South India. I had trusted her like a biological sister and had truly loved her with all my heart. Over the two years of therapy, I realised that perhaps she did not understand me due to differences in our upbringing, even though we both came from the same tribe. However, as a 19-year-old in 1997, I endured untold emotional pain, sleepless nights, and spells of crying because of her careless gossip, which was based on her imagination and assumptions about me rather than facts. Deep down, I knew that not all girls were the same, but the deep pain stayed with me. Somehow, I could never fully bring myself to completely trust another female friend.

While I had been blessed with a few wonderful girlfriends after that incident, it was in Lovily's house, while crying my heart out, that a healing process began in my heart. I felt liberated that I could cry in front of another human being without being judged or told that I was weak. It felt like I had come home after a long and arduous journey.

One of the reasons I never wanted to confide in others about my struggles was that I felt judged by my mum. Throughout my tween and teenage years, my mum, despite not meaning to, often made me feel guilty whenever I cried or tried to confide in her about my disappointments and pains of growing up. I know she meant well when she told me to be strong, that self-pity is unhealthy, that we must trust in God, have faith, and not be weak, but I began to take it literally. I believed it was indeed weak to cry whenever I faced difficulties. So, for many years, I lived without releasing my pain, living with aches and ailments in my body, without learning to express my anger or sadness, and without processing any of the traumas I had experienced while witnessing my mum and her siblings deal with mental health issues.

I had learned to shut off my emotions very early in life. Year after year, experience after experience, trauma after trauma. By the time I experienced my final breakdown in 2007, my emotions had become extremely toxic. Going for therapy for two years was like going for a long detox programme. Some days, I stayed in bed, staring up at my dorm room ceiling. Other days, I experienced amazing love, grace, and empathy from my friends and professors at BUSTH that made me feel my feelings of uselessness and helplessness were being washed away.

One such experience was an encounter with Professor Glen Messer in his office. I had signed up for a church history course taught by Prof. Messer during the spring of 2008 but was unable to finish my weekly reports despite making my best efforts. I had trouble concentrating and was left with no choice but to request more time and permission to submit my reports later. To my utmost surprise, Dr. Messer asked me questions, listened to me, and made me feel at ease about my struggles with depression. He told me that I was not alone in this struggle and that many others struggle with mental health issues. He asked me about my hobbies, so I mentioned a few, starting with watching movies.

I will never forget what he told me next, because it made me realise that my mental health struggles did not define me as a person and that there are people who truly understand mental illness. Dr. Messer exempted me from writing my weekly papers and attending his classes and instead told me to go and watch movies every week during his classes. I was shocked at his unconventional way of being a good Professor by treating me like his friend. He had seen the quality of my earlier reports and knew that I was a capable student. He asked me to only write and submit my final term paper. I went back to my dorm feeling humbled and truly relieved. The pressure of having to always be a perfectionist was lifted. I felt understood and cared for.

Every Tuesday during the spring semester of 2008, I would either hang out on campus or go watch movies at a theatre not far from the East campus of Boston University. Because of this gift from Dr. Messer, I learned to enjoy my own company, be true to myself, and appreciate the small things in life that we often take for granted. I still enjoy watching movies by myself to this day although I also love watching them with my family and friends at times.

For those struggling with depression, I would say that even if professional help is not accessible or available, it helps a great deal to find a mature and experienced person who is willing to listen and provide support. This is particularly helpful when facing panic attacks, feeling disoriented, or experiencing fear. Having a trusted friend to hold our hand can make a world of difference.

"A friend loves at all times."

Proverbs 17:17.

CHAPTER 11

Understanding Mental Illness

"For God has not given us a spirit of fear, but of power and of love and of a sound mind."

2 Timothy 1:7.

I lived in fear that mental illness was nothing but demon possession, due to witnessing my uncles and aunt (my mother's youngest sister) who never recovered sufficiently to live normally again. Although two of my uncles received some psychiatric help and were on medications intermittently, my aunt never received any help. Counselling or therapy wasn't even considered because, in the 1980s and 90s in Nagaland, there were no counsellors, as far as our family was aware.

In late 1991, my parents brought my aunt to live with us because she could no longer live alone. She wasn't getting along with her neighbours, and we saw her anger directed at practically everybody. Having grown up being loved and cared for by her, it was deeply confusing and painful to see her lash out in anger at her loved ones, including me, and accuse us of imaginary things. This was particularly bewildering as I was entering my teenage years, already struggling with confusion, and trying to cope with many challenges as a sick girl.

It wouldn't be an exaggeration to say that, at that time, there were no resources or help of any kind in Nagaland to deal with mentally ill patients or support families struggling with a mentally ill person.

Neither the church nor society seemed kind enough to offer support and love. When I was about 17 years old, a guest preacher at our church mentioned my grandfather's family in his sermon. During a Sunday evening service, he claimed that because my grandfather (whom he knew), a former Baptist pastor, had changed his denomination to the Nagaland Christian Revival Church (NCRC), and so God had punished his family by letting three of his children go mad. By then, my parents had moved from our small town to Dimapur city, and the preacher was unaware that we were present while he used my mother's family as an example.

What he didn't know was that my grandparents had started attending the Christian Revival Church because of a Prayer Centre called Chathe Prayer Centre, run by the Nagaland Christian Revival Church. This Centre had taken in my first uncle (who had lost his mind) and my mum's other siblings out of sheer compassion. The church reached out in love, prayed, provided shelter, and supported my mother's family without making them feel judged. Even though my two uncles lost all sense of normalcy, my mother, her other siblings, and my grandparents experienced a profound change in their understanding of grace and unconditional love. They faced immense pain, judgement, shame, and helplessness, but God used this Prayer Centre and church to extend grace and unconditional love to my mother's family in their time of need.

In narrating this incident, I am not passing judgement on our existing Baptist churches. I am still a member of the Sumi Baptist church in the small, beautiful village of Vihokhu, in the suburb of Dimapur, and I will continue to strive to create awareness about mental health and wellness with the knowledge I now possess. I am also pleased to see many churches, organisations, and hospitals joining hands to reach out to those struggling with mental health issues. We have come a long way, but there is still much more to do in educating and equipping ourselves to help those in need of support.

Years later, when I began my pursuit of theological education, I was able to contemplate deeper, read and research more on mental illnesses, the causes of mental disorders, and the struggles of others who had dealt with mental health issues. I met many fellow depressives while in Boston, and slowly but surely, I realised that help is available if we are willing to seek it. I am still educating myself and learning as I go along about mental illnesses and disorders. What I am certain of is that anyone facing mental illness needs healing of the mind, body, soul, and spirit. They need much love, deep empathy, and understanding of their helplessness, as well as all the support they can receive without feeling like they are a burden.

I also believe that lay people in the church need to be educated and made aware of how a person's brain and body are affected by depression or any mental disorder. My desire is for the church to encourage its congregation to seek psychiatric help, therapy, and counselling, alongside reaching out with prayers for those facing panic attacks, anxiety disorders, and other severe mental health challenges. Even if the prayer team recognises that anxiety, worry, and fear can be attacks from the enemy of our souls, the appropriate response is to hold the hands of those seeking help and let them know they are not alone – that God is with them in their anguish and pain. Judging those who are already broken only makes them feel more condemned, isolated, and worthless. People struggling with brokenness are often judged as having less faith which is like rubbing salt into someone's wounds. Instead, letting them know that God is with them in their brokenness, loving and accepting them, can help them realise that God truly loves them.

Some of the things one may find helpful in facing and dealing with mental health issues are listed and explained below:

1. **Understanding Our Patterns**: From my personal experiences, I had no idea I was so mentally unwell, even though I had carried emotional wounds, sadness, and grief for many years. I didn't realise that my fears, anger, inability to let go, and trust

issues stemmed from the traumas I had faced. These traumas had affected my brain, causing my mind and thoughts to react a certain way whenever I encountered emotions that reminded me of past painful experiences. I seemed to have no control over my emotions, which would overwhelm me and drag me back into deep depression. I would remain in a state of shock, fear, denial, or anger for days, endlessly rehashing events, questioning why they happened, how they could have been avoided, and ultimately blaming myself, feeling that life had no meaning.

For days, weeks, and months, I could only see things from a negative perspective. It would take months, sometimes even a year, for me to slowly detach from those strong emotions. However, I would end up facing the same difficult situations related to my studies, interpersonal relationships, or cultural experiences. When I finally admitted that I was tired of suffering in silence and sought hope through therapy, I began to identify the situations and experiences that triggered my depression. I realised that, just as exposure to extreme cold, rain, or heat could cause physical reactions, our inability to express anger, process pain, or deal with uncomfortable emotions could affect our brains and bodies in the long run.

Through therapy, I understood my pattern of self-blame for every mistake, my inability to let go of negative emotions, and my constant fear of disappointing myself. I realised the need to let go of certain people and unpleasant memories and to protect myself from unhealthy situations. Most importantly, I learned that I couldn't control everything, and that finding peace required me to let go and move on. Therapy helped me see that my control issues were not beneficial and that trying to manage every outcome in my life had only led to more disappointment and hurt.

As I learned to let go of many emotions, I found comfort in seeking help from friends, appreciating myself for enduring emotional pain, and pursuing higher studies abroad. Listening to sermons and messages from Christian speakers who had overcome their traumas by believing in God's Word and allowing Him to heal their wounds was also immensely helpful. Breaking the cycle of self-harm due to my inability to forgive myself for wrong decisions took a lot of courage and practice over more than a year.

Being kinder to myself was encouraged by my therapist and new friends who reached out to me during those years. Coffee dates and lunch outings with Katie Garcia (now Sage), window shopping and enjoying Japanese noodles with my dear friend Hee Jin, and hanging out with Tonia Petty regularly brought me joy. By the summer of 2008, nearly a year into therapy, I could genuinely say that life was beautiful. There were still painful and dark days, but I was much more aware that I wasn't alone in my sadness, loneliness, and suffering. I knew my life mattered not only to God but also to my family and many friends who appreciated me.

I began to find meaning in my suffering by allowing myself to be vulnerable with a few female friends, who ministered to me, cared for me, and supported me. It was comforting to have girlfriends who genuinely wanted to see me happy, whole, and healed. Life seemed to be just beginning for me in the summer of 2008. Though I was 30 years old, I felt as if my youthful years were just starting.

2. **Triggers**: My panic attacks usually occurred when I felt I couldn't meet the expectations I had set for myself academically. It was incredibly liberating to realise that my worth as a person is not dependent on my grades or performance. Discovering this in my late twenties was painful because, throughout my

life, I had tried to please my parents and extended family by proving my worth through academic achievements. Although I hadn't done too badly, already pursuing my third master's at a prestigious university in America, I couldn't stop berating myself whenever I received a poor grade. My obsession with academic excellence was akin to an addiction. The more I stressed about my grades, the more broken I became.

Once I gained this realisation, I slowly began to take pride in my resilience. I had survived years alone at South Korea, balancing a part-time job with a demanding graduate programme while managing my health issues. Finally, I could acknowledge the challenges I had faced without letting them deter me from pursuing higher education. These realisations did not come about suddenly but emerged over many months of painful therapy sessions with Dr. Goodman, who patiently helped me work through layers of unprocessed emotions. I had always felt shame, regret, and anger over my inability to graduate at the top of my class for my previous degrees, despite starting well. Letting go of this expectation was both liberating and painful.

I had to mourn the loss of my dream of academic laurels and wake up to the fact that I was a student at Boston University, a well-respected institution, living in a city where I met top-notch researchers, well-known clergy, world-class professors, business executives, artists, and creative people almost daily, even while riding the train to my classes. This realisation was beautiful and one for which I am deeply grateful.

By the summer of 2008, I was also working as an Administrative Assistant to the Executive Director of the Boston Theological Institute (BTI), a respected theological consortium in the greater Boston area and North America. My role with Dr. Rodney Petersen, the then Executive Director, and the

Assistant Director, Dr. Marian Simion, allowed me to interact with many clergy, professors, and researchers from esteemed churches, organisations, seminaries, and universities. I assisted in coordinating workshops and seminars with respected scholars, particularly in areas of Religion and Conflict Transformation/Peacebuilding.

One of the most memorable experiences of working with Dr. Petersen was organising the 40th Anniversary celebrations of BTI at the Harvard Divinity School on the Harvard University campus, attended by presidents of renowned seminaries, theological and divinity schools from North America. Despite continuing my weekly therapy sessions and still experiencing dark days, I felt I was doing something worthwhile. I put my networking and clerical skills to use and learned about social justice and peacebuilding while meeting incredible people. Although I berated myself for not winning academic awards, I felt fortunate to be surrounded by world-class theological educators and administrators. I felt small, like an ant, among so many renowned professors whose books are read worldwide, but I was humbled that someone as broken as me could still find enough healing to pursue what I had worked so hard for.

3. **Acceptance:** The human heart is deceitful, as the prophet Jeremiah wrote in Jeremiah 17:9: "*The heart is deceitful above all things and beyond cure. Who can understand it?*" For many years, I tried hard to hide how deeply I was hurting. It was my pride and inability to accept that I was completely broken without the help of God and my friends. I began to realise that many people had allowed God to help them deal with their pride and were living fruitful lives, unafraid to reveal their vulnerabilities to trusted friends. Slowly, I was able to accept that I was completely helpless on my own. The realisation that I was mentally and emotionally unstable felt like a stab to my heart. I had clung to the belief that I was

strong, unbreakable, and capable of anything. Looking back, I felt foolish for not wanting to seek help, even from a friend who could have offered a shoulder to cry on. I had relied only on myself, which did not serve me well.

A part of me still felt conflicted about admitting that I was desperate for help, yet another part of me felt relieved that I had hit rock bottom. I realised that the only way I could truly live again was to seek whatever help was available. Facing, feeling, and admitting my absolute helplessness in even getting through the day brought more pain. However, being able to admit to myself and to others that I was very sick and needed help set me on a path of discovering God's deep love. I was a broken human being who desperately needed a saviour, one who not only forgives the sin of pride but can redeem and restore all broken lives and dreams.

4. **Finding a Support System:** Although I knew there were support groups for addicts and terminally ill patients, I wasn't well-informed about mental health and wellness to realise that I could find a good support system for myself. As I have mentioned throughout, God, in His wisdom, began to bring friends into my life who, during the spring and summer of 2008, were quite comfortable discussing their struggles with depression, addictions, suicidal tendencies, and terminal diseases. Some of them prayed with me over the phone and in person on a weekly basis. A younger friend named Heidi Cochran, a trained nurse and an amazing evangelist, whom I met in Yonkers, New York, during the summer of 2008, became a constant source of support over the following year. She would call me every week to check on me, cheer me up, encourage me with her incredible stories of complete dependence on God, and end our phone conversations with heartfelt prayers. This truly built me up.

Although Heidi and I are no longer in touch, I will forever remain grateful to her for being a willing vessel of God and showing me His love in a very tangible way. I know her reward in heaven will be great for using her God-given abilities and time to invest in a broken and needy youth.

5. **Finding Resources and Using Them:** Until I arrived in Boston and friends noticed my struggles and encouraged me to seek help, I had no idea that resources were available. I had no hope that a life like mine could ever be restored. Now I know that there are online resources to educate oneself, support groups, counselling centres, mental health clinics, and more. Admitting to ourselves that we are mentally and emotionally unstable is a bitter pill to swallow, especially for those of us who like to keep everything under control, or at least try to fool ourselves into believing we do. However, once we understand that mental and emotional illnesses are just like any other illnesses, we will be better prepared to seek psychiatric help, therapy, counselling, etc.
While social media can contribute to mental instability and addictions, there are also many support groups on social media with content in both audio and visual formats that can help educate those struggling with despair, depression, suicidal tendencies, and more. We can make use of these resources to help ourselves and others.

6. **Commitment to Remaining Positive:** Even though it is impossible to think clearly enough to establish any regular healing practices during a major emotional or mental breakdown, I now make a conscious effort to feed my mind with positive thoughts. I know that I must try to replace negative thoughts with positive ones by reading and listening to uplifting and motivating messages daily. Meditating on the Word of God, maintaining a daily routine of reading or listening to Christian speakers who preach faith-building

messages, and staying in touch with friends who pray for me all keep me aware that I am not alone in my faith journey. The simple belief that we are alone can lead us into a deep and dark journey of loneliness and sadness.

Choosing to focus on God's goodness, surrounding ourselves with friends who keep us grounded and rooted in the Word of God, who build us up and encourage us, are the best ways to avoid deceptive thoughts that life is meaningless and useless.

> *"The Lord is my light and my salvation—*
> *whom shall I fear? The Lord is the stronghold*
> *of my life—of whom shall I be afraid?"*
>
> Psalm 27:1.

Section 3: Embracing the Future

Wrong Thinking Equals Wrong Results

CHAPTER 12

True Partnership

"But the fruit of the Spirit is love, joy, peace, longsuffering, kindness, goodness, faithfulness, gentleness, self-control. Against such there is no law."

Galatians 5:22-23.

On December 11, 2009, I married a man that God had been preparing for me for years, and He was also preparing me to become his wife. My husband, Major Dr. Mughavi Sema, pursued me during the two-and-a-half years I was in America studying. It has been nearly 15 years since we got married, and God has proven to me that He is faithful and keeps His promises to His children. My husband has been God's instrument of love to me and an answer to my prayers. I am reminded year after year that God knew exactly what He was revealing to the prayer lady about my future husband on that lovely autumn afternoon in South Korea when the Holy Spirit allowed her to minister to me about him. This side of eternity, I feel most blessed to be loved and cared for by a man of integrity who fears the Lord.

Our marriage has not come about without its share of stories, events, sacrifices, adjustments, and compromises from both of us. I have had to put all my peace-building theories and skills to use to make this marriage a partnership that God intended it to be. Most importantly, it is the deep love of Jesus Christ that has bound us together through all our life's experiences, because Jesus is our true and only foundation. My relationship with my husband is based on mutual respect and admiration. While we are different in many ways, we bond over our love for food, comedy, and meaningful conversations on issues and topics of mutual interest. We were both raised by very godly and prayerful mothers, and it has been my greatest privilege to see my husband transform into the man of God he is today.

By the time we got married, we had both matured emotionally, having experienced life in multicultural settings, struggling in foreign countries as international students, and facing the challenges of navigating life as young people. I honestly did not know what to expect of marriage. In fact, the idea of being married was terrifying to me for most of my early adult life. So, everything we have built together until today has been filled with pleasant surprises at most times and some shocking revelations about each other at other times.

While I am a Naga woman, very proud of my identity as a Sumi tribal woman, raised by a very conservative, godly mother, I also lived in two different countries, studying and working as an independent woman who made her own choices for daily life. Even before I went abroad to study, I taught at a Bible college in South India at the age of 24. Therefore, having to live and coexist with another human being on a daily, weekly, and yearly basis took some time for me to get used to. In hindsight, the reason my husband and I now have an ever-growing, healthy relationship and beautiful partnership is because we have been able to respect each other's space, value each other's gifts as well as our own areas of expertise, and retain the ability to appreciate each other's differences. While we have had a few major arguments over the course of our marriage, I can honestly say that most of the hard decisions we have had to make have been done with prayers and waiting upon the Lord, and without being disrespectful to each other.

I am grateful that I married after having worked on myself, learned to value myself as God values me, and truly understood that I cannot expect my husband to be someone that only God can be to me. While I respect, admire, and love the man my husband is, I know that he cannot be my source of fulfilment, which only Jesus can be to me spiritually and emotionally.

During the first seven to eight years of our marriage, I had no interest in helping with my husband's business enterprises, even though I ardently prayed for all his projects and ventures. My understanding of business and money was that they were secular and not sacred enough for a theologically trained person like me, who was called only to preach and teach. Then, in 2016, my mother gifted me a devotional book by Os Hillman titled "Today God is First (TGIF)." My mother always gifts devotional books to her loved ones at the beginning of each year.

Over the course of that year, as I read the devotional book daily, my eyes were opened to the fact that the gospel is needed in the marketplace as much as, if not more than, it is needed in the church. Jesus taught in synagogues, but He also walked the dusty roads of Palestine and preached to people wherever He met them. The sad thing is that I had previously heard, participated in workshops, and read about Business as Mission, taking the gospel to the marketplace, and that every vocation is a calling. Yet, it took me a year to understand that every born-again disciple of Jesus Christ has a calling and a commission to preach and make disciples of all nations, which definitely includes the marketplace. I began to realise that God had allowed me to marry a businessman for a reason, even though I had believed that my husband was the exact antithesis of me.

I had gone to study at a Bible college at 18 and had studied Theology throughout my youth and adult life. I was raised to believe that everything involving money also involved greed and sin. I often promised myself and even told my friends many times that if I ever married, it would be someone who had studied like me and had a vision to teach, preach, and pursue academics seriously. So, when all circumstances, prayers, and directions led me to marry my husband, I surrendered to being led by God, knowing deep down that He was bringing us together for a purpose. I had no idea how God was going to transform my misconceptions and lack of knowledge about His involvement in every area of our lives. Year by year, God revealed His wisdom to us as we continued to let Him lead us. It has been nothing short of a miracle to witness God's abundant blessings in our personal lives, experiencing His presence in our relationship with each other, and in the lives of friends and family.

My husband studied medicine at Kharkiv National Medical University in Ukraine, but he is more of a businessman than a medical doctor. He is a very committed, sincere, and hardworking man with great work ethic. He was commissioned into the Territorial Army (TA) of the Indian Defence Force in 2004 as a Lieutenant. Since the TA is a voluntary reserve force of the Indian army, it is meant for citizens who are already employed in mainstay civilian professions. While the TA officers have a part-time commitment, the benefits and honour are as good as those who serve full-time. As a result, ever since we got married, I have had to live alone (and now with our three kids) for two months every year while he goes for his posting.

As of 2024, my husband has retired voluntarily for two years now. He was last posted in the Andaman and Nicobar Islands (Indian Ocean) with the 154 Battalion of the Bihar Regiment. Over the past few years, I have seen God work through my husband, deepening his knowledge of the Word of God as he became actively involved in the Gideons International Ministry. While I have had to put my academic dreams on hold to raise our children, God has been teaching me about complete dependence on Him, waiting upon Him, and realising that, ultimately, everything is about Him. There have been many moments when I felt overwhelmed and very disappointed by the responsibilities of being a mother and a wife, especially having to put my dream of pursuing doctoral studies on hold and being at home every day. However, I have also learned to enjoy cooking, planning and executing my children's birthday parties, and hosting friends and family for dinners and BBQs – activities I could never have imagined doing when I was busy studying and planning academic pursuits.

I have taken up gardening as a small hobby, set up a small home-based nursery where I sell exotic fruit plants and flowers. Tutoring our three children with their after-school assignments has also kept me busy. My mother and I co-founded a small faith-based NGO in 2009, a few months before my wedding. Our NGO is called Kupukini Women Society (KWS). We reach out to down-trodden women by providing skill-oriented training like soap making, and beading. KWS organises workshops and seminars on Mental Health and Wellness, Organic Gardening and Basic Floral Designs for women in and around our city.

My husband and I are often asked by young couples about the secret to our happy marriage. There are a few practical guidelines we have both adhered to ever since we got married. The most important thing I always mention is this: Jesus is the reason we are happily married. Had I married before God dealt with my pride, selfish desires, and personal ambitions, I wouldn't have lasted in marriage for even a week. Even though my husband truly cares about me, and I have so much respect and deep love for him, living with another human being is a lot of hard work. Having a loving personal relationship with Jesus has enabled me to view my marriage as an eternal covenant God allowed me to enter. My theoretical knowledge of biblical principles about unconditional love, patience, forgiveness, and peace has truly been tried and tested over the course of our nearly 15 years of marriage. I can say with conviction that Jesus is more than able to bless an earthly human relationship for His glory and conform us to His likeness if we are willing to walk in humility before Him and walk in love with our family members, choosing not to take offense even when human limitations hurt us deeply, offend us, and make us angry.

I look only to Jesus when I am disappointed or hurt because He alone loves everyone else with their limitations, just as He loves me with my human failings. I am only as strong as my dependence on Him is complete. Jesus is my only defender when I feel defenceless. The Word of God is my only shield against the attacks of the enemy upon my life and my family. Marital relationships are likely universal, but Asian culture is much more community-oriented than the Western world. Accommodating our in-laws, siblings, uncles, aunts, and cousins is expected. We also have social obligations, such as attending weddings, funerals, and visiting the sick, from our community, tribe, and clan, even if we don't have personal relationships or close friendships with them.

Despite being brought up in a very traditional Sumi Naga household and respecting all that my parents thought was important, I never quite understood their need to cater to everyone around them without thinking about themselves. Living unselfishly for others may seem godly and traditionally correct, but living only to please others, or out of fear of not being considered good enough if we don't please everybody, seemed overwhelming and tiresome to me. I feel blessed to be part of a church community and to have friends and family who are always there for us, just as we try to be there for them. However, the need to keep up appearances in Naga society seems to be increasing, even as materialism is spread into all spheres of life. Given that everyone I meet talks about the need for change in how we expect each other to behave, sadly, I see very few people making any effort to be agents of that change. That's why my husband and I have purposely set boundaries on social engagements, despite being criticised as selfish sometimes.

One thing I have been very conscious about is not to be pretentious to my husband's side of the family. I know that God sees my motives, secret thoughts, and intentions, which is why I constantly remind myself that my husband's family is my family, even though we come from different bloodlines. I vowed to treat all his relatives as I would treat mine, with equal respect, love, and generosity.

Every family has its dynamics, holiday traditions, ways of expressing emotions, and verbal communication methods. My husband and I have done our best to create an environment for our three children to be their own persons, express themselves politely but clearly, apologise and mean it when they hurt someone, and be sincere in every small task they are asked to do, including their studies. I still rely only on God's grace when I am sometimes harsh in trying to correct them. I am grateful for the grace that sustains me, turning my guilt into petitions and prayers when I know I am failing.

We pray regularly for our children to grow up to be all that God has created them to be. While I have hopes and dreams for their future, I know I will never force my children to live my dreams. While it is imperative that they excel in whatever line of studies or professions they pursue later in life, my husband and I pray that they will accept and know Jesus as their personal Saviour above all else. Jesus must be our rock on whom you and I must rely on, even for our children. Even when our children are misbehaving, we must trust the Holy Spirit to continue working in their hearts rather than focus or impose on them for a short-term behavioural change. For me, I need to sometimes remind myself, that they are God's children first before they were ever ours. Our greatest desire for our children should not be that they have a high-paying job, but they hear and follow the leading of the Holy Spirit. All other blessings will follow.

> *"Therefore humble yourselves under the mighty hand of God, that He may exalt you in due time."*
>
> 1 Peter 5:6.

CHAPTER 13

Mental Health and Spiritual Warfare

"Now may the God of hope fill you with all joy and peace in believing, that you may abound in hope by the power of the Holy Spirit."

Romans 15:13.

Growing up, I was very confused about how to differentiate between a person who was possessed and someone who was mentally ill. Thankfully, the awareness and conversation around mental health issues have significantly improved in my home state of Nagaland and across India since my childhood. Today, we have many professional counsellors, psychotherapists, clinical psychologists, and psychiatrists working alongside NGOs, hospitals, and mental health advocates to create awareness and provide support and resources to families and individuals dealing with depression and various disorders. Celebrities in India have also been shedding light on mental health issues they face under the public eye and constant scrutiny. However, the need for awareness and education remains great and urgent. There is also a pressing need to integrate wholesome spiritual practices with seeking medical and counselling help for those struggling with mental health issues.

Although I am not a trained counsellor or mental health professional, my desperate need to understand, educate, and empower myself in the area of mental health and emotional disorders led me to sign up for an elective course on 'Depression and Dark Night of the Soul' in the autumn of 2008 at Andover Newton Theological School. The course was taught by Dr. Britta Gill Austern, a renowned professor of Clinical Psychology. The course was intense, with challenging readings and papers to write, but I learned that depression and disorders have troubled people since the beginning of human existence. Growing up, I watched my relatives deal with severe mental illnesses, and witnessed my mum's family cope with shame and untold emotional and mental anguish, but they never really talked openly about it. I thought we were alone in this struggle. The feeling of isolation is real and deep because we are unable to express our feelings of shame and the depth of emotional hurt that we encounter when we see our loved ones losing their sanity and becoming mere shadows of their former selves.

I witnessed my aunt, who was an accountant, lose her mind year by year. She had started working early and lived alone for many years by the time I went to live with her to attend a school close to her house. I stayed with her for three and a half months in 1991, when I changed schools mid-year. I was 12 years old and in the seventh grade. I knew she loved me, and she took good care of me, but one day, she started raving about how her siblings and I were disrespectful towards her. To this day, I do not know what triggered the outburst. There were a few more episodes when she would suddenly start crying and saying strange things that I did not understand. I also noticed that she spent most of the night awake, praying silently. Because my aunt was a God-fearing woman who had been actively involved in church activities, serving the church for many years, I never doubted the sincerity of her faith and prayer. Later, as I grew up, I realised that she was already in deep trouble during the months I lived with her. She had stopped attending church, cut off ties with her friends, and was practically alone. She stopped working after experiencing some problems at her workplace. She was living in complete isolation. It saddens me now when I think about my twelve-year-old self living with a very disturbed woman in her thirties. I had no idea what she was dealing with back then because I was entering my teenage years and was facing many frustrations, confusions, and questions of my own. Moreover, my mother, who was living about 26 kilometres away from the town where my aunt and I were living, had no idea that her sister was slowly losing her mind.

Almost two decades later, as I started to understand the symptoms and patterns of people dealing with depression and disorders, I felt very sad that my aunt did not receive any help during those years when she was still able to function. I remember a particular Saturday morning when she started singing loudly right outside her house, and the whole neighbourhood came out to look at her. I was very embarrassed, but I had no clue that she was dealing with anger and depression that had been left unattended.

As I grew older, faced my own fears, struggled to come to terms with my desperate need for help, read up, attended courses, and educated myself about how our brain and body react to trauma, injustice, and painful situations, I began to better understand PTSD, panic attacks, anxiety, clinical depression, bipolar disorder, addictions, schizophrenia, etc. The more healing I received through therapy and the support of friends and by educating myself, the more I felt a sense of obligation to spread awareness about the importance of taking care of our mental and emotional well-being. I had not been taught that unresolved grief, unresolved anger, the inability to express our voices and opinions against injustice we have suffered, dealing with chronic illnesses, etc., can affect our brains, altering the way we relate to others and behave. It is now common knowledge that if depression goes untreated, it can alter the brain. We must also understand that depression impacts the body and our physical health, causing many issues like digestive problems, migraines, extreme fatigue, and body aches.

I was privileged to complete a certificate programme on Religion and Conflict Transformation at Boston University through the BTI. Since I worked at the BTI with Dr. Petersen, coordinating with divinity and theology school students, including chaplains, pastors, rabbis,

Restorative Justice practitioners and students from other schools at Boston University, I was encouraged by Dr. Petersen to explore peacebuilding and theology, the role of religion in peacebuilding, and similar topics. For this, I remain very grateful to him. As part of the programme, I took a course with Dr. Shelley Rambo on Trauma and Theology. This class introduced me to neuroscience and allowed me to learn about how the chemicals and neurons in our brains react when we experience extreme loss and grief, the different stages of grief, and how human lives and our faith journeys are greatly impacted and forever altered by the traumas we face.

I want to quote Dr. Shelley Rambo from her book *Spirit and Trauma: A Theology of Remaining*, because her writing truly reflects all that I have experienced in my brokenness. She writes, "Language falters in the abyss; it fractures at the sight of trauma. We need to find a different way of speaking from the depths, reclaiming the notion that language about God is always fractured, always fractured and never complete."[6]

While these lines may sound like there is no hope for resurrection, I know for a fact that I was dragged down to that abyss and stayed there for nearly two years because of the traumas, the aftermath of those stinging, shockingly painful years that my family and I experienced over two decades. Even though God orchestrated all the events that led to my years of finding help spiritually, emotionally, medically, and psychologically, and helped me experience resurrection in every sense of the word, I know that many have not survived trauma and continue to live in that endless cycle of pain and brokenness. This is the reason I am sharing my story – that while we have the resurrection of Jesus that is ours too, this resurrection experience can be extended to those who need it if we as believers become more aware that we can be agents of Christ who can help broken people see and experience life after death.

Yes, faith is required to pursue the path of God, but love is the greatest force that can allow a person to find hope to want to live again. Showing the love of Christ and extending hope to a person who feels

---

[6] Rambo, Shelley, *Spirit and Trauma: A Theology of Remaining*, Westminster John Knox Press, 2010.

worthless and useless, and who feels that their life is meaningless and purposeless, will take more than preaching and praying. Yet, we give up so easily on ourselves and even more easily on others. The good news is, God never gave up on me. That is precisely why I now know that I should never give up on those that the world and even the church sometimes give up on, and that may include family, friends, or people in the church or our workplaces.

All I knew earlier about people losing their minds was that it was demonic possession and that there was nothing much we could do except to exorcise the demons. So, being introduced to these courses truly opened my eyes to my own ignorance about how unanswered questions about pain, suffering, and our relationship with God can and should be addressed, even though we may not get all the answers we want in ways that we want to. Even though I had studied Liberation Theology and knew in theory about the concept of freedom and liberation and had heard and read about the freedom we have in Christ, I experienced liberation from ignorance that caused me decades of pain. Slowly and painfully, I began to learn to let go of the shame, embarrassment, and deep wounds I had carried in my heart ever since I was a little girl, who cared enough to see and feel the pain I saw my loved ones go through. Letting go of all my hurts, anger, confusion, and so many other unexplainable negative emotions against God and against people who had held my heart, soul, and body captive took me over two years.

I was often mentally exhausted, but by the end of 2008, I was slowly able to reclaim parts of myself that I thought had completely died. It would not be wrong to say that I began to like myself again, which felt nice. I once posted a message on my Facebook page that I was in love with myself. It may have come across as being narcissistic, but I was finally able to see myself through the eyes of God, realising that I am loved by my maker and that it is okay to fail sometimes or many times. By then, I knew that God would never give up on me—He never had. Truly understanding that I am created in God's image, that while every aspect of my whole being felt fragmented for exactly a decade, I had always been loved by God. I had always been blessed with a loving family and friends who truly cared about me, and it felt like waking up after a very long, bad nightmare. A very deep sense of gratitude replaced all the negative thoughts that had plagued me for so long. I wish I could say that this transformation happened overnight, but God had to deal with every aspect of my thought life and my faith life one by one. Though it took two years for me to feel like a reborn person again, I was so glad to have been on a journey that involved being transformed in every way, one step at a time.

The path that I thought I was headed on, the kind of life that I thought I would be living, and the Christian ministry that I thought I would be involved in are not exactly what I had imagined as a very enthusiastic 18-year-old who was starting her theological training. I have evolved, I have changed, I have been transformed, and I have literally been resurrected from spiritual, emotional, and mental decay, - for real and from the inside out. While I feel more like my true and old self, I can also say that I am not the same person I was, however contradictory this might sound.

I am still a student of mental health and wellness and certainly not an expert on matters of religion and medical science. However, I believe that our spiritual enemy, the devil first attacks our thoughts because every part of our life stems from our thoughts. I also believe that the name of Jesus is more powerful than any other name in heaven and on earth. I believe that deliverance from the attack of the evil spirit is possible in the name of Jesus. However, I am also very convinced that for a person dealing with depression to find restoration and the feeling of ever being made whole again, the incorporation of faith and prayer, a strong emotional support system, medication, and therapy are all equally important. I know that many struggle with emotional and mental illnesses and never fully recover or find healing even with all the help they receive. For those people, my heart aches. I wish I had all the answers and, in many ways, writing this book is one way of reaching out to those who are still struggling as I did. Perhaps my story will help a few to know that they are not alone, that they can and must seek help, and that there is hope and certainly a light at the end of a long, dark tunnel if one is willing to do the work needed to find healing or a new way of life.

In my case, realising that I am not alone, and that mental illness is like any other illness, many others suffer from and struggle with was the first step towards feeling a sense of normalcy about seeking psychiatric help. The second liberating step was learning that the mental breakdowns I experienced every few years were not my fault. The next painful step was learning to consistently go for therapy, take my medications regularly, and stop beating myself up every time I felt weak and vulnerable or when I slipped into some of my old habits, especially hurting those who cared about me. In retrospect, I realise that I would not have felt so isolated and alone had I been able to confide in someone sooner about my confusions, fears, and doubts while I was growing up. Instead, I did the opposite by suppressing all my angst and feelings and became so good at acting that I ended up being a phoney. It was a very sad realisation when it finally dawned on me that I had been thinking the wrong way, treating myself the wrong way. I was pleasantly surprised to learn that I deserved better because Jesus had provided a way for me to live without self-condemnation, as found in Romans 8:1; *"Therefore, there is now no condemnation for those who are in Christ Jesus."*

Most of all, the Word of God sustained me in ways I never imagined, even though in theory, I had studied God's Word so much. The writer of Hebrews 4:12 says, *"For the word of God is living and powerful, and sharper than any two-edged sword, piercing even to the division of soul and spirit, and of joints and marrow, and is a discerner of the thoughts and intents of the heart."* This verse sums up the work God did in my life as I allowed the Holy Spirit to minister to me many times by reading the Word of God and meditating upon the very Word that became flesh in Jesus Christ.

"Blessed be the God and Father of our Lord Jesus Christ, the Father of mercies and God of all comfort, who comforts us in all our tribulation, that we may be able to comfort those who are in any trouble, with the comfort with which we ourselves are comforted by God."

2 Corinthians 1:3-4.

CHAPTER 14

Motherhood

"God is our refuge and strength, a very present help in trouble."

Psalm 46:1.

I am a mother to three very active children who seem to be growing up at lightning speed. On August 16, 2011, my husband and I were blessed with a healthy baby girl. During the first trimester of my pregnancy, I craved Korean food and mangoes. Since it was winter in India and not mango season, I would calm my cravings by plucking mango leaves from our tree, crushing them with my fingers, and smelling them. To satisfy my craving for Korean food, I made homemade Kimchi using available vegetables.

Since I did not experience anything serious throughout my pregnancy, I thought I was going to have a very easy delivery. To my greatest horror, I had to go for a C-section a day and a night after I was first induced for artificial labour because I had no pain even though my expected date of delivery was due. I had not prepared myself mentally or emotionally for extreme physical pain. I was very hopeful that I would have a very easy and normal delivery. However, as I waited to have a normal delivery, my daughter became distressed and was not breathing when she was taken out. My mum later told me that my daughter had turned blue and did not make any noise when the doctors first took her out. The doctor and nurses had to do everything they could to make her breathe, and she was kept in the NICU for three nights. I was physically exhausted and even more traumatised emotionally. My legs and thighs were badly swollen before the C-section, and while I had no regular labour pain, the discomfort in my tummy and inability to breathe well did not bode well. I also experienced severe back pain. After it was clear that I was not going to be able to deliver, I was wheeled into the operating theatre. I remember how tired I was. I was in the ICU for a night for observation after the C-section. Thankfully, I was shifted to a private cabin the next day, where I spent a week in painful recovery.

The physical pain and the sadness at not being able to feed the baby as much as I wanted were also distressing. Because of the way my body had been stretched to its limit while trying to have a normal delivery, I felt very tired and worn out. When the painkillers wore off, I was in so much pain that my whole body would sweat. Since it was mid-summer in India, the discomfort of physical pain combined with heat and humidity was unimaginable, even with the air conditioner on. I had never imagined that I would go through so much suffering again. It is never easy to go through surgery. The stitches were removed on the eighth day post-C-section, and I returned home. The baby kept me busy after that.

Now, my life revolved around my daughter. Despite the physical discomfort and sleepless nights, my baby brought my husband and I so much joy. I named her Eva, and my husband named her Totikali. 'Toti' in our dialect means 'girl', 'Ka' means 'rule', and 'Li' is usually a suffix used for feminine names. Her official name is Eva Totikali and she loves baking, crafting and is now a certified junior coder. We lovingly call her Toti, and her friends and teachers at school know her as Eva. She is a very determined girl who gives her all to anything she sets her mind to. She can basically train herself in pretty much anything she is interested in. During spring of 2024 Eva developed a simple app and won first prize at a coding competition her school participated in. She represented her school along with some of her school mates. She will be turning 13 years old on August 16, 2024, but is already quite tall and wears shoes bigger than mine.

Taking Eva to the paediatrician for her monthly vaccinations was painful to watch for the first few months, especially as she cried after receiving her shots. With time, I began to realise that it is okay to allow our children to experience pain, for them to realise that we will always face pain and challenges as long as we are alive in this world. I am still learning how to help my children respond to painful situations and it is always a challenge.

Back in 2019 a missionary friend advised me, "Boka, do not worry too much about your children getting bruised or hurt. Let them fall and make mistakes because that is how they will learn to take care of themselves." I still have trouble allowing my kids to run around, scream, and jump, fearing that I am not protecting them enough. I am also a work-in-progress, and I know that while I will do all I can to protect my children in whatever ways I must, I should also remind myself that God is my children's ultimate keeper. I trust Him to protect my children, guard them, and guide them, even though I may not be physically present with them all the time.

God, in His wisdom, allowed my body to rest for a few years and blessed us with a second baby, a very healthy son, on December 22, 2014. Since God had blessed us with a daughter, I had prayed for a son, and God in His faithfulness blessed me with two sons in two years.

When I was pregnant with my first son, during my first trimester (the third month), I started to bleed one Sunday. Fear crept into my heart and thoughts. I called my mother and told her to start praying that I would not lose the baby. I went to the doctor and was given some medication and advised complete bed rest. For the second and third trimesters, I was very careful to follow the doctor's advice by not going anywhere and resting at home. God in His mercy allowed me to carry the baby to full term. We named our middle child, our first son, Tokupu Seth.

Seth loves mathematics and numbers. He is a very quiet boy, often lost in his world. He started talking at 15 months, and by the time he was a year and a half, he conversed with us like an adult. Sometimes, I joke that he is a man trapped in a boy's body. We are so grateful to God for our son Seth.

Although I did not experience morning sickness or any specific cravings while expecting Seth, I did crave sour food and lime juice. Luckily, I had a few lime plants that bore many fruits that year, allowing me to drink fresh lime juice every day until the end of the year. I knew I would not be able to have a normal delivery because I did not feel normal throughout the pregnancy. The Word of God kept me focused on the finished work of Jesus Christ for my wholeness and healing.

One day, towards the end of my pregnancy, I started to feel overwhelmed at the thought of enduring so much physical pain and discomfort. I decided to spend some time in prayer and couldn't help but cry out to God, asking Him why I had to go through so much pain whenever I felt I had already suffered enough in life. Amid my tearful prayers, I suddenly started to sing the hymn "Lest I forget Gethsemane, lest I forget thine agony, lest I forget thy love for me, lead me to Calvary." Although this was a hymn I had always loved singing, I had not been thinking or planning to sing it when I started praying. The Holy Spirit ministered to me as I sang this hymn through my tears. I knew in my spirit that while Jesus had paid the price for my salvation, sicknesses, and complete redemption, I felt comforted knowing that Jesus understood my sufferings and that I was not alone even when I felt abandoned. Even though I knew that sickness and pain of any sort were not from God, He could still use my sufferings to draw me close to Him, to engulf me in His love. The physical suffering, emotional torment, and spiritual alienation that Jesus endured at Calvary to redeem me from sin and curse made so much sense to me. The Holy Spirit comforted me, assuring me that even in my darkest days, Jesus is with me. His presence was so real that afternoon that feelings of self-pity and the question of "Why me?"

were completely gone by the time I finished praying. I can honestly say that encouraging others in Christ has become much easier for me after that experience because I know that Christ is truly with us in our sufferings and that He understands our sorrows and heartaches.

Looking back at my younger years when I feared marriage and motherhood more than anything else, I am amazed at how a very strong-willed woman like me has weathered many storms of sleepless nights, long days with sick and grumpy kids who are noisy, jumpy, and hungry at all times, needing my attention. While there are days when I wish for more quiet time, there are many more days when I am so grateful for the kisses and cuddles, hugs, and 'thank you' I receive from my loving children. They extend so much grace to me that I cannot help but feel God's love being extended to me through my children. Like many mothers we hear our children telling us "You're the best mom in the whole wide world," which brings us comfort knowing that they accept and love us with all our faults. When I hear my children appreciate me it brings a warmth to my heart. I can never thank our heavenly Father enough for granting me the privilege of being a mother.

> "The righteous cry out, and the LORD HEARS, and delivers them out of all their troubles."
>
> Psalm 34:17.

CHAPTER 15

Trusting in God's Hand

"My help comes from the LORD, Who made heaven and earth. He will not allow your foot to be moved; He who keeps you will not slumber."

Psalm 121:2-3.

In April 2016, I began to feel unwell daily. My face broke out, I lost my appetite, I felt nauseous most days, and I didn't want to be around people. I knew it wasn't depression because I was a grateful mother to energetic toddlers. Our daughter was in kindergarten, a curious little girl who came home from school very excited every day. Our son Seth was exactly a year and three months old. My hands were full.

Like many life-changing experiences, I had no idea I had conceived. I have been a thyroid patient since my mid-twenties, so I thought my hormones were acting up. My sister Ruth, a practising nurse who had gone on to do an MBA in healthcare, suggested I get a pregnancy test. I was unprepared for another difficult pregnancy and didn't expect her guess to be correct. To my shock and surprise, I found out I was expecting. While I was very grateful to God for the gift of life I was carrying again, the road ahead seemed difficult and burdensome.

My back hurt, and I couldn't move around much. Thankfully, my feet did not swell this time. The strangest thing that year was that God allowed me to cross paths with several women and young girls struggling with deep depression and anxiety. The first was introduced to me by a mutual friend. This educated lady from a good family was struggling with severe anxiety, which broke my heart during our first meeting.

I had never sought to counsel people, but encountering these emotionally and mentally needy sisters felt like God bringing us together for healing. I am not a certified counsellor as I have mentioned before, but God in His wisdom allowed me to take many counselling courses during my theological studies. My personal emotional and mental struggles have also given me a sense of authentic empathy for those struggling with emotional and mental issues. Since I do not have a counselling practice, I met this lady once a month at my house and talked over the phone for a year. We also became good friends, for which I am very grateful. When she asked about my fees, seeking to pay me, I declined as I did not feel it would be ethical to receive payment. I genuinely wanted to help a sister in need of love. The love and friendship I have cultivated with those seeking my help have been more valuable than any monetary payment.

Reaching out to brothers and sisters suffering from emotional and mental issues during my third difficult pregnancy kept me focused on others' sufferings rather than my own. I now understand what the theologian and priest Henri Nouwen meant in his book, "The Wounded Healer"[7] – that we can be agents of healing by giving ourselves and our services to the wounded even while we are experiencing brokenness ourselves.

During the nine months of waiting for my third baby, God also allowed me to minister to a very wounded girl for eight months. My heart broke for her because she was so wounded in her heart, spirit, and soul. I had to depend on the Holy Spirit during our interactions because she did not know who she was and constantly asked questions I could not answer. We had breakthroughs when we talked and prayed

---

[7] Nouwen, Henri J.M., *The Wounded Healer: Ministry in Contemporary Society*, Random House Publishing Group, 1979.

together, but there were many times I felt helpless in not being able to change her self-image. It was not my duty to fix her, and all I could do was direct her to the One who created her, loves her deeply, and wants her to enjoy life to the fullest.

About three weeks before my due date, I went to my gynaecologist for a regular check-up. He told me that my amniotic sac was drying up and that I needed hormonal injections every eight hours for a week. It was not pleasant getting injected every eight hours. After a week of injections, I consulted the doctor again, and he scheduled a C-section for the next morning, which was a big relief. I went home and packed for the trip to the hospital. The next morning, I was admitted.

At some point during the day, I was taken to the operating theatre. The routine felt so familiar to me that I was not fearful about the surgery, even though I was not looking forward to life after another C-section. This was my fourth surgery after marriage, including an appendectomy in 2012, just after my daughter had turned a year old. The anaesthesiologist had been the same for all three previous surgeries. This time, I was pleasantly surprised to see a petite lady anaesthetist. She seemed pretty shocked that I was coming in for my third C-section. She told me I was brave to have two C-sections within just two years. While I knew that C-sections were not particularly pleasant, I was unprepared for the depth of pain my body would have to endure again.

On December 3, 2016, our son and third child, Athikivi Jabez, arrived. The date coincided with my parents' wedding anniversary. To this day, our son Jabez celebrates his birthday with his grandparents, who celebrate their wedding anniversary. Jabez weighed 3.5 kg (7.7 pounds) and did not make a noisy entrance into the world unlike his older brother, who had cried loudly in 2014. I was awake and aware of everything around me throughout the C-section because I was not given general anaesthesia.

After I was wheeled out of the operating theatre to the recovery room,

I could not sleep, despite trying. As the anaesthesia slowly started to wear off, I began to experience extreme pain around my back and abdomen. I motioned to one of the nurses in the recovery room and told her that I was in pain, to which she replied that it is normal for a patient to be in pain after surgery. I was unwilling to tolerate so much physical discomfort. Since the nurse was not very understanding, I told her that this was my third C-section and that I needed a painkiller. She seemed shocked that I had had two C-sections in two years and became more sympathetic. She also told me that her sister had three babies through C-sections. She immediately gave me a painkiller through an IV (intravenous), but it did not seem to work. About four to five hours later, I requested another dose of a painkiller. This time, they gave me a shot via IM (intramuscular), which seemed to help.

I do not quite remember how many days the baby and I spent at the hospital, but I remember very clearly that it took me nearly three months to feel any sense of normalcy even after going home.

Thankfully, Jabez was a very quiet baby who did not cry unless he was wet, hungry, or thirsty. I remember spending many days and nights crying while lying in bed because I was so sick and tired of being in so much physical pain and discomfort. I have always been very good at hiding my pain from my loved ones, so I remember my husband being shaken and shocked when I cried in front of him once. I am sure he won't remember the incident even as he reads my recollection here. Every bone in my body seemed to ache every day, and I longed to feel fresh and light. There was a heaviness in my body, a huge burden in my heart, and a deep sadness that I did not seem to be able to shake off, which continued for a few years.

During the spring of 2017, I went for a master's health check-up at a hospital. I wanted to make sure that my health was normal because the aches and pains continued. Thankfully, everything seemed normal except for some deficiency in my bones when I had the bone density test done, for which I was prescribed calcium supplements. However, the constant pain on the left side of my back, which went all the way down to my left thigh and knee, troubled me a great deal. So, while on a trip to Bangalore in the summer of the same year, I went to another hospital and consulted a good neurologist who told me I had no problem and prescribed me antidepressants. The medication made me very drowsy, and as I had a baby who was not yet a year old, I decided not to continue with the medication.

There are days when the enemy tries to intimidate me with lies, telling me that I am not in control of my children's futures and that, no matter how hard I try, I will never be able to protect them from harm and danger. But I know better now than to believe his lies. I know that the God who delivered me from the darkest pit is the God who created my children. God loves my children more than I could ever love them. I know that the creator of the universe, the God of all gods, the King of Kings, is the lover of my children's souls. Nothing comforts me more than the thought that God knows all the days that were ordained for my children before one of them came to be (Psalm 139:16). I know God will take care of my children as He has promised in His Word about never leaving us nor forsaking us.

> *"He gives power to the weak, And to those who have no might He increases strength."*
>
> Isaiah 40:29.

CHAPTER 16

Victory Over the Battle

"My flesh and my heart fail; But God is the strength of my heart and my portion forever."

Psalm 73:26.

In mid-September 2019, my husband encouraged me to get an ultrasound from a gynaecologist because I was overweight and my tummy was bloated. Friends often asked if I was expecting again, but I had a tubectomy during my third C-section and knew that wasn't the case. I was unpleasantly surprised to find out I had a large ovarian cyst on my right ovary. The doctor informed me that this type of cyst is known as a 'chocolate cyst' and explained that the only permanent cure for this condition, caused by endometriosis, was to remove my ovaries. Since my husband was away on his annual military duty, I requested conservative treatment for a month or so. The doctor prescribed a hormonal medication to suppress the cyst's growth.

A month and a half after starting the medication, my mother-in-law passed away at 97. She was a powerful woman of great faith, a godly and prayerful woman who had raised my husband, his two brothers, and two sisters with much prayer and obedience to God. Although we miss her presence, God comforted us in knowing she had gone to meet her Saviour, Jesus, whom she faithfully served and loved until her last breath. She left behind three blessed and accomplished sons, two blessed daughters, several grandchildren, and a few great-grandchildren.

My mother-in-law, the late Mrs. Shiyili, and my husband's sister-in-law, Mrs. Hokali, were instrumental in encouraging my husband and me to get to know each other better. I remain grateful to our loving Father, our great and merciful God, for granting me ten years with my mother-in-law. Her prayers still sustain her family. I feel blessed to be a part of her great legacy of faith and work. After she passed, I remembered the many prayers I had prayed as a single girl, asking for godly in-laws. Truly, God answered my prayers by allowing me to marry a man whose mother was a woman of great faith.

Four days after my mother-in-law's passing, my aunt (wife of my paternal uncle, V.V. Chishi), whom I lovingly called Iza Khetoni, also went to be with the Lord at 63. Unlike my mother-in-law's funeral, where there wasn't much visible grief, my aunt's funeral was emotionally intense and painful for me and our family, perhaps because her death was unexpected. Despite the grief, I needed to follow up on my cyst. So, a day after my aunt's funeral, my husband, sister, and brother accompanied me to a neighbouring state to see a reputed lady gynaecologist, recommended by a friend. She advised me to undergo an ultrasound and a biopsy. The scan showed that my cyst had reduced in size drastically, and the biopsy result was negative. I was advised to stay on medication for three months and return for a review.

When we returned home to Nagaland, I had no idea of the ordeal that lay ahead in the coming months.

Fast forward to 2020. I was busy looking after two school-going children and a toddler. I did not have much time for myself, though I was on medication for my ovarian cyst. My husband and I had been constructing our farmhouse away from the city since 2019, and we were planning to move bit by bit. I have been blessed to have relatives and hired help to assist in caring for the children and doing household chores. However, I have realised over the years that nobody can replace a mother in her children's lives. I am grateful to God for providing me with an environment, resources, and situation where

I can be a stay-at-home mum, even though I have longed to work full-time many times. I remain grateful every day for a husband who works hard and provides well for his family.

There have been many times over the past 13 years when I have felt useless for not being able to work, teach, travel, and pursue my personal interests. At times, I have felt like I have wasted my education, for which I put in many years of hard work. However, God in His mercy and kindness has always granted me peace about staying at home for this season of my life, which seems to keep getting stretched year by year. I have also wondered if this season of staying at home will ever end. Still, deep down in my heart, I know that I am where God wants me to be, which has brought me much comfort when the enemy tries to tell me otherwise.

In mid-February 2020, my husband and I travelled to Bangkok, Thailand, to attend the wedding of a family friend's daughter. When we were returning home at the end of February, the Wuhan Virus that famously became known as Covid 19 had spread to Italy. We had read that a Thai traveller had tested positive, and I remember coming back to India with a feeling of unease. Surely enough, by March, India already had many Wuhan Virus (COVID-19) patients, including in our neighbouring state of Assam, where I had gone to see the lady gynaecologist.

Even though I was scheduled to meet my doctor after my last visit in November 2019, I could not go because the borders were being sealed due to the spread of this deadly disease. I did not think much about my cyst since I had finished three months of medication, and I thought I would be okay. We had started to move our belongings to our farmhouse bit by bit, every week. My husband remained at the construction site and I kept going back and forth, packing from the old house and unpacking at the new house. The road to our farmhouse was not good at that time, and anyone who has visited our part of the world will know that in many rural areas, good roads are still a distant dream.

By the end of March and beginning of April, the very first phase of lockdowns started. A week after a day-long lockdown was imposed, the government decided to implement a partial lockdown, allowing vehicular movement for only half a day.

Two days before Good Friday of 2020, as we were trying to unpack some boxes at our new farmhouse, I began to experience a great deal of pain in my abdomen. I was bloated and felt very uncomfortable. My youngest sister Ruth, a competent nurse (no longer practising), and my husband were around. I consulted them and took some painkillers to ease my pain. By Thursday morning, my sister wisely took me to the hospital. We consulted the doctor who had done the ultrasound. She told me I had ascites; a condition wherein abdominal swelling is caused by fluid accumulation. It turned out that my cyst had burst and was causing the fluid to accumulate. Since we couldn't go out of the state, I was admitted to Olive Hospital, which was not far from our old house. I had gone to the gynaecologist there in 2019 and had first found out about the chocolate cyst. The same doctor advised surgery without much delay. I was told to get admitted the next evening, which happened to be Good Friday. We drove home very slowly and, the next day, we packed, preparing to go to the hospital, even though it was Good Friday. We left for the hospital in the afternoon and I was admitted for pre-operative procedures. Even though I did not look forward to another surgery, I did not fear going to the Operation Theatre the next morning.

I was advised to undergo a full hysterectomy and honestly thought and expected that this was going to be my final trip to the hospital. I was wrong. Of all the surgeries I had undergone in the past, this was going to be the most extensive and challenging one. Since all my previous surgeries had taken not more than 45—60 minutes, I went into the Operation Theatre thinking I would be done within that time.

When I regained consciousness a day later, I tried to open my eyes but couldn't. I felt tired and sleepy, and my tongue felt like a dry leaf. The surgery had taken place on a Saturday, and I felt a little more awake by Monday afternoon. I was told that the surgery took four hours and that I had lost a lot of blood. This was because I had adhesions from my previous surgeries that had to be scraped off before the doctor could remove the cyst, my right ovary, and the uterus. I was also told that the doctor decided to keep my left ovary since it was healthy and I was losing blood.

Although it was unpleasant to feel pain and discomfort, I felt relieved that I was on my way to recovery. I also thought I would not have to visit the hospital as much anymore. I did not know that my hospital visits were going to increase even more after the surgery. Even though I felt very weak and tired, with every part of my body aching, I had the most amazing and comforting experience on the second day after my surgery. As I mentioned earlier, I could open my eyes on Monday afternoon. I could drink a bit of liquid and use the restroom on my own.

I don't remember the exact time, but it was early evening when I felt cold and sleepy. I remember my husband pulling a thin blanket over me. I fell asleep and immediately had the strangest dream about crossing a small river, with dense forests on both sides. I saw a group of people rowing boats, and I was in a boat too. From a distance, I could hear the most beautiful hymn-like song being sung by a choir. The song was so beautiful, and the dream seemed so real that I could remember the tune and words of the song for over a week after waking up. In the dream, I crossed the river and reached a large area that seemed like a conference space with different rooms. In my dream, a woman named "Saori" welcomed me and introduced me to many missionaries and pastors, many of whom I recognised as Koreans. Saori told me she was German, but I thought she looked part-Caucasian and part-Native American. I woke up and realised I had been dreaming. I must have been asleep for a short time, but I felt much more refreshed. I couldn't get the dream out of my mind and noted down the name Saori on my smartphone. After being home for a week or so, I tried to google the name Saori. Interestingly, I found out that 'Saori' is a Japanese word meaning 'colour of sand' and is also used as a girl's name in Japan. When used as a feminine name, Saori translates to 'beautiful fabric,' 'white floating lily,' and, most beautifully, 'blossom.'

It has been four years since my surgery, but I cannot forget the dream. I believe God used that dream to comfort me and remind me that He is indeed a master weaver, the ultimate designer of my life.

The pain in my abdomen was excruciating during my four-day stay at the hospital. On the fifth day, I was allowed to go home. Since I couldn't travel far to our farmhouse, my sister looked after me at our old townhouse while my husband and extended family members, including my parents and cousins, cared for my three young children at our new farmhouse.

A week later, I returned to the hospital to get the stitches removed and then moved to the farmhouse to be with the rest of the family. I couldn't move around much, even though I tried to walk a little after my small meals. It took almost a month for the pain in my abdomen to completely subside. The children had their online classes, and there were lockdowns and partial lockdowns, but I needed to rest, so I had to consciously refrain from doing any strenuous work around the house, even though I desperately wanted to set up everything around the new house. I had time to think, read, and pray, even as the world seemed to have come to a complete halt. I had much to reflect upon and be truly grateful for, being alive after having had brushes with death so many times. I should mention that the nurse who assisted my doctor during the surgery happened to be a distant relative. She told me that my pulse rate dropped significantly and they had to use chemical cardioversion to restore the rhythm of my pulse. I had wondered why my tongue felt so dry and the extreme fatigue persisted until two days after the surgery. Later on, I learned that the medicine used to recover the pulse rate caused side effects, one of which is dryness of the tongue and mouth.

I had been thinking for quite a few years about writing a small book on the many occasions that God had healed me supernaturally since I was a youth, but I had procrastinated. However, as I had a lot of time to myself during this recovery period, I felt that I should start writing without any more delay. So, I decided to write a few paragraphs or pages every Saturday, starting in May 2020. Everything seemed to operate in slow motion, and life seemed so much simpler with everyone staying home, and extended family members not being able to visit each other. This period was the first time in the 11 years of our marriage that my husband had enough time to stay home and practically do nothing except look after his animals and plant some more trees at our small farm.

I thought I was recovering very well over the next two and a half months, but, in mid-July, I suddenly started to experience severe pain in my abdomen. I couldn't digest any food, solid or liquid. At first, I thought it was gastritis. Since most hospitals were sealed off due to COVID-19 being at its peak in our part of the world, my husband and I both thought it was safer for me to be treated at home.

A few days later, it became clear that something was wrong with my abdomen because the pain prevented me from sleeping at night. I was in constant pain throughout the day. My sister was in touch with a medical specialist because we all thought I was suffering from acute gastritis. I couldn't retain even water. As soon as I consumed any food or liquid, I had to use the toilet. On the advice of the doctor (via phone calls), my sister injected me painkillers, which would help for about an hour or two at most. There are no words to describe the kind of pain and torture I endured this time. It felt like a heap of burning coals and hot ashes were being heaped inside my stomach continuously for three weeks.

There were times when I wondered if I would ever be free of physical pain in my body. I had my sister Ruth taking great care of me during the day and my husband staying up with me till late at night, but I had to fight the battle of pain with every ounce of strength I possessed. I couldn't lie down for too long because the pain was too much. If I gulped water, I couldn't pass gas, which was torturous. My sister, who had been a nurse in the ICU at a reputed Christian hospital in Nagaland, began to suspect I was suffering from a terminal illness like stomach cancer.

After the house turned very quiet at night, I would get up from bed and walk around the room, praising God, and lifting my hands in prayer. I couldn't walk straight, so I bent while walking around our dark bedroom. I didn't want to wake my tired husband. Even though the pain was inexpressible, and my stomach felt like acid was being poured all over it, deep down in my heart, I had enough reserve of God's goodness such that I didn't allow myself to feel any self-pity. I constantly spoke of life and healing over my organs, my cells, and my body, even though it felt like my body was being destroyed. As I look back now, I realise that having a doctor husband and a very good nurse as a sister was God's way of proving to me that He knows exactly what I need. I am so grateful to my heavenly Father for being very personal to the extent of knowing exactly what I needed when I needed it, and who I needed.

On August 12, 2020, I told my husband and my sister that it was best I went to the hospital since medications at home were not helping me. So, despite our worries about COVID-19, after exactly three weeks of intense pain and drastically losing about 10 kgs of weight, my sister and I went to the hospital where I underwent surgery. I met the doctor who advised an endoscopy and a CT scan. The results showed that I had minimal gastritis and an umbilical hernia. My sister heaved a sigh of relief when she saw the reports. The doctor advised me to be on complete bed rest, a very soft diet, and to never lift any heavy objects. I returned home with the hope that I would be able to digest liquids at least. Thankfully, for the first time in three weeks, I had porridge at my parents' place and did not have to use the toilet right after eating.

I had much time to think, reflect, and pray during those three painful and traumatic weeks. Those were very dark nights indeed. If not for the Holy Spirit ministering to me and the reserve of God's word in my heart, I am sure I would not have survived a few nights, let alone three weeks of complete, utter darkness. I would have been crippled with fear with thoughts of dying and wanting to give up on life because I had seen enough physical pain, mental anguish, and emotional agony to last me a lifetime. During every season of pain and struggles, I see and experience God's strength and ability to sustain me, and this season was no different.

I decided to give up on medications and painkillers, instead, I fasted and prayed at home for divine intervention. Deep down in my heart, I knew and believed that God can raise the dead and that there is no sickness that the blood of Jesus cannot heal. On August 17, I started to fast and pray till 3 p.m., continuing until August 21. I knew I had nothing to lose and much to gain by seeking God in prayer, even though I was physically weak. During the first two days, I experienced extreme pain in my stomach every now and then, such that I had to lie on the floor, writhing in pain in between prayers. However, I was committing my physical limitations to God, the limitations of medical science to God, and trusting Him to heal my body. I truly believe and know that by the grace of Jesus, I am healed as seen in the scriptures (Isaiah 53:3).

On the third day of the fast, I realised that the extreme pain was decreasing in both intensity and frequency. Even though my body still felt weak, my spirit felt lighter, and I could sleep at night.

By the fourth and fifth days of my fast, the severe and excruciating pain completely left my stomach and my whole body. Praise the Lord! Hallelujah!

I first saw in my mind's eye that I was completely healed, even as I kept praising God for the blood of Jesus that was shed to heal my broken body. Despite the crippling pain and the constant fear of darkness and death that tried to take hold of me in those three weeks, especially during those quiet nights when all my loved ones were asleep, God allowed me to have complete victory over sickness, darkness, loneliness, and pain. During my five-day fast, I was greatly comforted by reading the 77th chapter of the Psalms over and over again. The Holy Spirit reminded me of the countless times when He had comforted me, literally held my hand, and healed my body. My heart was filled with deep gratitude to be alive so I could tell the world about the miracles that God has performed in my life, just as He has been doing since the creation of the universe.

When I first started studying at Bible college, all I ever wanted was to pursue God's purpose for my life and live it out, no matter what it took or where it led me. I was very enthusiastic about sharing with others what God had done in my life, the miracle of experiencing the healing of my nose bleeds for over a decade. As I progressed in my theological studies, exploring various methods of studying and doing theology, I somehow began to idolise scholars, academics, books, programmes, and Christian ministry. Yes, I prayed and attended church, spoke, and taught in churches and seminars. I shared whatever resources I knew of with other brothers and sisters who needed guidance. I was even involved in reaching out to the downtrodden and the marginalised by setting up a non-profit organisation. I did not know that a stronghold still existed in my mind about the need for worldly recognition, the need to feel validated by fellow Christian ministers as worthy of being appreciated as a well-educated person. In theory, I knew that Jesus left the splendours of heaven to walk the dusty roads of Palestine, minister to needy people, and die on the cross for someone like me. It was not that I was ungrateful for the gift of salvation; I was and am truly grateful for the saving knowledge of salvation by grace through faith. However, the Holy Spirit gently reminded me that Jesus loves me, would still love me, and could use me even if I did not have any theological education. He knew me and He loved me. This simple reminder, as I prayed during those five days in my bedroom, brought me a sense of freedom and made me realise that it was truly about having a very intimate relationship with Jesus.

The joy of knowing Jesus as my Saviour, my healer, my best friend, my brother, my portion, and my everything, cannot be compared to anything this world has to offer. This joy of knowing Him is the reason I want His love and His power to save and redeem to be made known to everyone I come across for as long as I breathe. I want my life to touch others' lives, my knowledge of God and His Kingdom to be imparted to whoever I cross paths with, and I want the world to know that Jesus heals every sickness. Jesus can heal and restore our broken bodies, our wounded souls, and spirits, and He is more than willing to save, deliver, and heal everyone who is willing to come to Him. I have faith and belief in medical science as a wonderful gift of God to mankind. I also know that when medical science fails or has limitations, God's power to heal and restore is available to whoever is willing to trust God as the only source that can do what human beings cannot.

My life is a testament to the fact that when every thing fails, Jesus never fails. He has proven to me multiple times that He can heal my body, mend my broken heart, restore my sanity (literally), and give me the power to live in victory daily, over every challenge the enemy throws my way. Even as I write this, I am on medication for another cyst on my only left ovary, for which I may need surgery. I am often asked if I face any fear when I am being wheeled into the Operation Theatre for surgeries. I have also been told that I am lying to say I have no fear, but I can confidently say that fear does not control me anymore. Even though it took me many difficult years to realise that fear is a spirit, I am not confused in any way that the devil loves to intimidate God's children with fear all the time. Timothy 1:7 reminds me clearly that God did not give me a spirit of fear, but a spirit of love, of power, and of a sound mind. I have the spirit of Christ living inside of me, which is why I am filled with love, and I have the power of resurrection in my body and spirit. Most importantly, I am not tormented by the lies of the devil that I am worthless, that my life is not worth living. My life is worth living, my time on earth is precious, and I intend to live a life of intention, one that will live out all the purposes God intended for me before the foundation of this world.

More than anything else, I want to proclaim the love of Jesus and His power to resurrect.

> *"For I will restore health to you and heal you of your wounds,'says the LORD, because they called you an outcast saying: This is Zion; No one seeks her."*

Jeremiah 30:17.

CHAPTER 17

Breaking Free

I wrote this book with the intention of reaching out to anyone living in bondage with the message that there is freedom in Christ. My greatest desire is for everyone reading my story to know that in Christ there is freedom from every kind of bondage. It could be fear, lack of self-esteem, pride, anger, extreme selfishness, disorders, painful past, hidden sin, and unforgiveness, or narcissism that is holding you back from walking out the plans God ordained for you while you were being formed in your mother's womb as David wrote in Psalm 139:13, *"For You formed my inward parts; You covered me in my mother's womb."*

God doesn't ask us to surrender our lives to Him because He wants to enslave us. It is because He wants us to walk and live in liberty that only Christ can offer us through the power of the Holy Spirit. As Scripture says, *"...I have come that they may have life, and that they may have it more abundantly."* John 10:10.

I was bound by fear and lived in complete bondage for ten long years. I was terrified of what people thought of me to the point of wanting to hurt myself because I loathed myself. I had an intellectual understanding that Jesus died for my sins, but I believed the lies of the enemy that I was not worthy of being loved and accepted because I was not perfect. I lived in defeat, completely bound in my mind. My decision-making and relationships were influenced by the enemy keeping me bound with his lies. I had been completely deceived to feel and think that I needed to be perfect in all ways, in the sight of everyone. I did not believe with my whole heart that God's grace was sufficient for me. My need to be perfect drove me to a place of complete darkness.

Even though I was a student of theology, preaching, teaching, and leading in worship, I felt like a phoney because deep down in my heart I did not fully trust that God could deliver me from my fears and darkness. I did everything I could in my power to feel strong, to be empowered. Yet all I kept feeling was a sense of great defeat, a sense of hopelessness without any sense of purpose in being alive.

But God in His goodness and mercy led me on a journey of healing and wholeness in ways I could never have fathomed, in ways only He could have orchestrated the healing process I needed to go through. Throughout the whole process of God's wondrous dealings with my trauma, my anger issues, my unusually dark sadness; my deep fear of trusting people even as I had to learn to stop beating myself up, God's grace never wavered. He kept showing me how much He cares for me by providing me with people I needed to be with, to learn from and to receive support. I had to be completely broken to be remoulded and renewed from the inside out.

Learning how to think new and positive thoughts instead of focusing on fear, doubts and mistrust, took me many years and I am still a work in progress. I had to commit myself to depend on God for every decision I needed to make. I learnt to stop depending on my own abilities to control my life the way I thought was best for me.

Little did I know that God is the greatest, the highest above all creations. He is the wisest, the most loving and always forgiving.

The more I started focusing on how good God is, the more I was able to let go of situations I cannot control. The more I let go, the more God showed me how faithful He is to those who put their trust in Him.

Goes doesn't care where we come from, He doesn't care how educated or not educated we are, how rich or poor we are, what mistakes we made, how sinful we lived. All God cares about is how precious we are to Him.

He is not only able to forgive us, but He is more than able to restore our health and the years that we lose to the enemy of our souls. He is able to give us new life, new habits and a new vision. All we have to do is admit to God and to ourselves that we are helpless without Him.

The road to recovery from depression, trauma, or from any kind of bondage is never an easy one. I know that instantaneous deliverance is also possible because there is nothing that God cannot do. However, our minds need renewal for us not to go back to our old ways of thinking and operating. That is why we need friends who will support us and hold us accountable. We need to study the Word of God everyday so that our old ways of thinking are replaced by faith in God's ability to restore us, renew us and deliver us completely.

If we take the first step and confess that we are helpless without God, He is more than able to lead us on a journey toward healing and restoration of the life we may have given up on. There is always a new beginning in Jesus because His love for us never fails. He never gives up on us. You have nothing to lose and everything to gain.

Try Him.

Let me pray with you...

Heavenly Father,

I lift up this precious soul who has read *Breaking the Silence* and now seeks Your healing touch. Lord, You are the God who sees all, the One who knows the depths of our pain and the unspoken struggles of our hearts. Just as You walked with me through my journey of brokenness and restoration, I trust that You will walk with them now.

Father, where there is despair, let hope rise like the dawn. Where there is fear, let Your peace calm every storm. Where there is pain, may Your healing flow abundantly, bringing restoration to their body, mind, and soul. Teach them to cast every burden upon You, knowing that You care for them more deeply than they can imagine.

Jesus, You are the Great Physician, the One who makes all things new. Touch the places in their life that feel too broken, too painful, or beyond repair. Shine Your light into their darkest moments, and replace their shame and sorrow with the beauty of Your love. Speak truth over the lies they may believe about themselves, and remind them of the infinite worth they have in You.

Lord, I also pray for the caregivers, families, and friends who walk alongside those who are suffering. Strengthen them with compassion, patience, and wisdom as they support their loved ones. May they reflect Your love and grace in every interaction.

Father, thank You for being the God who turns ashes into beauty, despair into joy, and brokenness into wholeness. Lead this person step by step towards the freedom and abundant life that only You can provide. May they feel Your presence, know Your peace, and trust in Your perfect plan for their life.

In the name of Jesus, I pray,

Amen.

God is Love

I look around me,
I see great beauty.
Creation, art, relationships.
I also see brokenness and ugliness.
Darkness of Sin.

The beauty of this world; in all its splendour.
Creation in all its glory.
Forests and jungles, flowers and bees.
Homegrown trees and beauty in the forests.
All beautiful to behold.

Happy faces, manicured gardens, and lawns.
Fancy four-wheelers, mansions galore.
Chandeliers, ginormous events.
Expensive houses of God booming.
God's people looking joyful.

I look beyond these beauties.
Beneath the surfaces,
I see the brokenness of hearts,
messed up lives.
Souls running helter-skelter,
In need of healing and restoration.

Tears shed unseen.
Regrets, confusion.
Questions: what could have been?
Shattered lives,
All these I ponder.

Only beauty cannot heal broken lives.
Gold and silver cannot redeem broken dreams.
A broken heart, a love lost.
A wounded soul, a lonely spirit.
None can heal.
Only Love can heal, repair, and restore.

Seek Love, Chase Love.
Never give up on Love.
Love will find us.
Love found me.
Let love meet you.

God is Love.
Bokali Chishi Mughavi

Everything Made Right

I sat in my dust and ashes
Numb in pain and despair
My head throbbing and heavy.
Confused, torn and tortured.

Endlessly weeping, never stopping.
Never being able to make sense of my losses.
Shaken to the core, writhing in deep pain.
Wondering if I would ever see a better day.

Anguish overtaking my heart
My soul crushed and in darkness.
Hope was nowhere in sight
Nowhere in sight for years.

Heavy heart, merely existing.
Never seeing any light of day.
No sign of change could I expect.
Only darkness and deeper darkness.

Alone, scared, fearful and angry.
Angry at myself, at my weaknesses.
Angry at my fears, regret that I was born.
My heart stuck in a very dark place.

Gloomy, achy heart.
Never at rest, forever seeking Love.
But did love even exist? I questioned.
Love didn't exist, I answered myself.

My heart roamed the streets of anger.
My soul tortured by demons
My legs weak, my body weary.
My Spirit completely broken and cast down.

Would anybody understand?
Did anybody care?
I did not think so, I did not believe so.
Because nobody told me I wasn't alone.

I felt all alone.
I suffered alone.
I sat in darkness alone.
Thinking I deserved to be alone.

Now I know better.
Nobody should suffer alone.
We all need each other.
We must reach out to each other.

Forgiveness awaits us.
Love that is patient
Ready to envelope us.
Ever ready, ever willing.

Radical Love, not deserving
Yet giving
Wholly accepted, everything made right.

Bokali Chishi Mughavi

Help Centres

LAPIYE Centre for Mental Well-Being

Toniho Complex Shop no 58
2nd Floor, opposite Green Park
Fifth mile, Chumukedima Nagaland
Phone number: +91 8730001800
E-mail: loviawomi56@gmail.com

OTHER MENTAL HEALTH SERVICES IN NAGALAND:

@DIMAPUR

NT-Revivify Counselling Service

KARIOS Counselling Centre

Fellowship Colony

JOYOUS LIFE: Professional Counselling Centre

@KOHIMA

Mental Health Mentor Counselling Centre
Mereima, opposite IG Stadium

State Mental Health Institute, Kohima

Centre for Integrated Counselling Services Kitsubozou,
near Panchayat Hall, Sector 5, Kohima.

TO LEARN MORE OR INVITE
BOKALI CHISHI MUGHAVI TO SPEAK

Contact Details

Email: kupukiniwomen@gmail.com

Facebook: Bokali Chishi

IG: chishibokali

INSPIRED TO WRITE A BOOK?

Contact

Maurice Wylie Media

Your Inspirational & Christian Book Publisher

Based in Northern Ireland and distributing around the world.

www.MauriceWylieMedia.com